Praise for

PERFECT MATCH

"Dr. Amy McMichael's *Perfect Match* delivers practical advice on how to secure a competitive residency position, as well as excellent advice for moving forward in your life and career, based on her thirty years of experience as an academic dermatologist, twelve years as a program director, eleven years as a department chair, and her own journey as a woman of color who consistently overcame systemic barriers and bias, large and small.

"This is a valuable guide for students seeking direction and for faculty committed to becoming more effective, empathetic mentors. One of the greatest take-home lessons of the book—whether to get a residency, to achieve greatness in your career, or to give back to your community—is to pursue your passion, which is exemplified by Dr. McMichael's passion for mentoring and its embodiment in this work."

STEVEN R. FELDMAN, MD, PhD
Professor of Dermatology, Pathology and Social Sciences & Health Policy
at the Wake Forest University School of Medicine

"*Perfect Match* by Dr. Amy McMichael is a game-changing guide that's packed with practical wisdom for building meaningful and impactful mentorships. Drawing from her own rich experiences, Dr. McMichael provides actionable advice for both mentors and mentees, highlighting the power of intentional engagement and introspection. This book is just as much about mentorship as it is about stewardship—inviting readers to take ownership of their own growth and well-being. In doing so, readers will strengthen their unique 'It' factor and contribute to shaping a more positive, empowering culture in medicine. This book is an absolute must-read for anyone passionate about becoming, or supporting, the next generation of physician leaders!"

BRIANNA DE SOUZA, MD, FAAD
mentee and colleague of Dr. Amy McMichael

"There is no one in our specialty of dermatology more credentialed to write this invaluable guide than Dr. Amy McMichael. While she has received every imaginable accolade for accomplishments in dermatology, it is her passion for mentoring learners that drives Amy every day. The readers will receive all of the precious pearls of wisdom that have been shared with countless young dermatology aspirants throughout Amy's distinguished career."

JOSEPH JORIZZO, MD, FAAD

Professor and Former Founding Chair of the Department of Dermatology
at the Wake Forest University School of Medicine

"*Perfect Match* is written by the *perfect* physician, my friend and colleague Dr. Amy McMichael. She is not only the *perfect* dermatologist, as evidenced by her exemplary accomplishments, but she is the *perfect* physician to write *Perfect Match*. Dr. McMichael cares profoundly for the next generation and has unselfishly, with joy and gladness of heart, mentored hundreds of underrepresented in medicine students. She always offers practical, well thought-out advice that is tailored to the individual student, all based upon her treasure trove of wisdom and knowledge.

"Dr. McMichael's commitment to nurturing future generations echoes the lessons imparted by our high school English teacher, Janet, who taught both of us to write skillfully and read analytically. Just as those teachings shaped our academic journeys, *Perfect Match* promises to equip readers with the tools to excel as candidates for dermatology residency."

SUSAN C. TAYLOR, MD, FAAD

Bernett Johnson Endowed Professor of Dermatology
at the Perelman School of Medicine and the University of Pennsylvania,
President of the American Academy of Dermatology (2025–2026),
and Founder of the Skin of Color Society

PERFECT MATCH

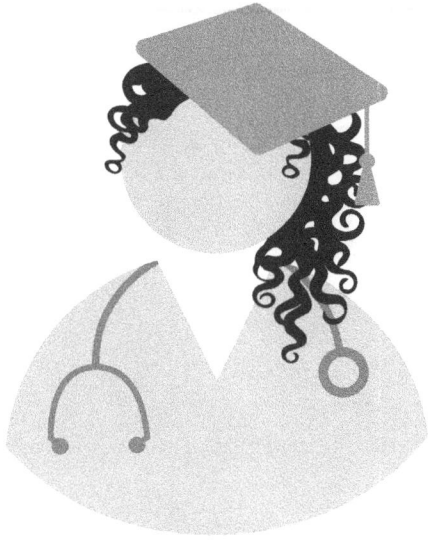

PERFECT MATCH

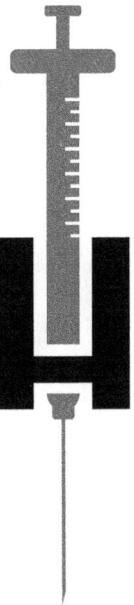

SECURE YOUR RESIDENCY SPOT & ACHIEVE GREATNESS IN DERMATOLOGY

AMY J. MCMICHAEL, MD

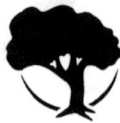

Published by

**MANDALA
TREE PRESS**
mandalatreepress.com

Paperback ISBN: 978-1-954801-94-3
Hardcover with Dust Jacket ISBN: 978-1-954801-96-7
Case Laminate Hardcover ISBN: 978-1-954801-95-0
eBook ISBN: 978-1-954801-93-6

MED017000 MEDICAL / Dermatology
MED024000 MEDICAL / Education & Training
BUS106000   BUSINESS & ECONOMICS / Mentoring & Coaching

Cover design and typesetting by Kaitlin Barwick
Edited by Justin Greer

dermdownload.com

*I dedicate this book to my mother and father,
who supported me unconditionally in my journey,
and to my husband, sister, and children for their
love and encouragement.*

"I rather think now, to tell the sober truth,
that it was merely my youth, first youth, anyway,
that was ending and I hated to see it go . . .
now I would have to go the distance."

JAMES BALDWIN
Nobody Knows My Name

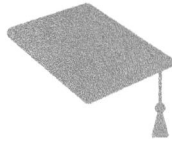

CONTENTS

CONTENTS

CONTENTS

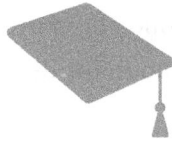

FOREWORD

By Dr. Shani Smith, MD, FAAD

LOSING OVER 80 PERCENT OF MY HAIR AS A CHILD WAS LIKE watching a part of myself slip away; it reached deep into my sense of identity. For a young girl, hair often plays a defining role in self-image and confidence. I remember staring into the mirror, feeling a profound sense of confusion and loss, searching for answers. This painful experience planted a seed of determination within me and ignited a dream: to uncover the science behind hair and skin so I could one day bring hope and healing to others facing similar struggles.

That dream carried me through years of rigorous study and ultimately led me to Dr. Amy McMichael.

Encountering her work in dermatology and hair loss, I knew I had found not only an esteemed physician but a mentor. She embodied compassionate expertise and showed me that true care involves seeing beyond the medical condition to the person behind the patient—their hopes, fears, and stories.

Choosing my medical school because of her presence was a pivotal decision, one of the best I ever made. Our professional relationship evolved into a friendship enriched by shared laughter, wisdom, and memorable moments—especially our good food experiences at conferences. In those moments, I learned that mentorship often extends beyond the mutual pursuit of professional achievements and can ascend to the discovery of one's purpose and personal fulfillment.

Dr. McMichael's guidance provided a grounded perspective, helping me develop my vision and sharpen my approach. Her insights, while occasionally different than my own, often challenged my thinking, allowing me to grow and evolve as a professional. I have always believed that my greatest limitations are the ones I set for myself, and her mentorship reinforced this belief, encouraging me to pursue my own path with confidence.

Many of you reading this have faced uncertainty and wondered about your future. Perhaps you have encountered challenges that made you question your direction or sought guidance from those you admire. I found valuable support during a critical phase of my journey, and you, too, may find someone who will illuminate your path and inspire you to pursue your goals.

The stories shared within these pages capture the reality of challenges we all may encounter, but they also underscore a greater truth: we are not defined by our obstacles but by how we choose to respond. Our decisions, actions, and determination shape who we become, turning hardships into opportunities. Therefore, empowerment lies in seeing challenges as catalysts for resilience, personal growth, and self-discovery.

My experiences have shown me that obstacles, though daunting, can become stepping stones. Success is not about avoiding difficulty but about facing it, adapting, and learning from it. As you delve into this book, I encourage you to reflect on the potential each story holds for transformation. You have the capacity to redefine your circumstances with determination and a solutions-oriented mindset.

This is only the beginning of your story. With guidance, perseverance, and a strong belief in your abilities, you have the power to shape your future and turn setbacks into success. Success is not limited to a select few; it's available to anyone willing to pursue it with passion, commitment, and an open mind. So, take that first step with confidence and embrace the possibilities ahead—your journey is yours to define!

Dr. Shani Smith, MD, FAAD
Chief Wellness Officer, Ashira Dermatology

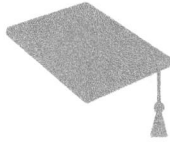

Introduction

MENTOR IN A BOOK

WHEN I DECIDED ON DERMATOLOGY AS A SPECIALTY OVER three decades ago, I was excited that I had finally found my passion in medicine. At the time, dermatology was a late match that was not determined until after medical school ended and during internship. When all my medical school classmates were opening their match letters in March of our senior year, it was discouraging to know I would have to wait until October to find out if and where I would match. But, at last, I opened the letter showing I had matched at my top choice at the University of Michigan—and I was over the moon. I had secured my best fit, and it set me out for a long and exciting career in the specialty of my choice. My hard work had paid off for the first leg of my training, and I knew that I wanted to pay it forward for others in the future.

For as long as I can remember, I have wanted to write a book that helps people see the world in a new way. This may sound strange, since I have already published over 160 scientific papers, written 12 chapters in textbooks, and served as an editor on 2 published dermatology textbooks. Don't get me wrong: I hope that everyone who has read any of my medical work has learned something new about dermatologic conditions . . . but I imagine that few have had a life-changing experience reading them.

That's why I'm writing this. *Perfect Match* is a comprehensive guide for the minoritized medical student who is grappling with how to be an excellent candidate for dermatology residency but is still struggling to succeed in rotations, research, and application preparation—likely because they feel like they don't belong.

I have developed this book to change the life trajectory of any medical student who needs help getting to the next level in their early training. These medical students are *good* but need help getting to *great*—and I want to stand in that gap. Ever since I started medical school, I have been appalled at how few books there are to prepare students for greatness. When it comes to applying to competitive medical specialties, there is little guidance other than checklists of tasks that should be completed in each year of medical school. These checklists are helpful, but I want medical students to have a true "mentor in a book."

Many students contact me because they need help showcasing their achievements and presenting them in a way that will garner a competitive residency in dermatology. I think some of them hope I have a magic sauce or secret that will get them to where they want to go. And every year, after the residency match takes place, calls and emails flood in from unfortunate applicants who did not work with me and who did not match in dermatology. My first thought is always this: *If only I had a chance to speak to them when they were early in medical school, I could have helped them.*

Some students who contact me are frantic to squeeze in last-minute research projects to add one small piece to their resume before their final applications. I am not the person for those students. I thrive when working with students who are willing to approach their time in medical school with a well-rounded plan. This is not a book about capturing dermatology as a prize—because getting into residency is just the beginning. The prize is moving through residency training successfully and giving back to the community with your practice of the specialty.

I don't have any magic, but I do have the experience to delve into accomplishments and to highlight where more work needs to be done. I am offering a book that puts more meat on the bones than the well-written medical student guidelines for competitive residencies. In my real life, I offer those students who contact me a short meeting (virtual or in person) to offer advice and a summary of how they can move forward successfully in their chosen specialty, especially for those who choose to apply for dermatology residency. These meetings have been a joy for me and, hopefully, helpful for the students.

Still, these meetings are short and not longitudinal for most. I want this book to be the longitudinal mentor to those who need that extra step up, that word of encouragement, or that confirmation to continue pursuing a competitive specialty like dermatology. This will be the companion to your in-person mentors. There are no promises of a successful residency match in this book, of course, but I *can* promise straight talk and many examples of how to shine as a medical professional. The real goal is to help you find

Find your place in medicine and feel comfortable in your skin while you're practicing.

your place in medicine and feel comfortable in your skin while you're practicing, thus leading to a successful career.

In this book, I will cover how to find a mentor and enhance the mentor–mentee relationship. But even if you already have fantastic in-person mentors, this book is still valuable because there are always new ways to look at preparing for residency. These stories and lessons explore different ways to be visible in the best way, find your particular brand of leadership, perform at the highest level, and handle failure more adeptly. I have also included practical advice for preparing your residency application, engaging in research while in medical school, prepping for interviews, writing a glowing personal statement, and improving your overall communication skills.

I have focused on dermatology because that's my beloved specialty, but it's my hope that college and medical students (and perhaps other learners) can use my experiences to guide them in times of need or help them recognize when to change their approach or step up their performance on the way to residency and beyond. These chapters give salient pointers to enhance the things that are in our power to control: preparation, performance, and dedication. With my experience in the specialty of over twenty years as a leader in academic dermatology, I aim to give learners a vision of what a committed and prepared physician looks like.

Speaking of outward appearances, my experience as a person of color in medicine has taught me many lessons. I constantly face microaggressions in the workplace, and I aim to teach other young physicians to recognize and handle these situations with professionalism and grace as they arise. This is one of the things we cannot change, but we can alter our approach and learn to allow our performance to speak for itself. Others may think of me and other physicians of color as "African American physicians" (or insert any other minoritized group instead), but I want those who read this book to know that they can be just "physicians"—and *great* ones.

Reach inside yourself and find the excellence that is there. Come along on a brief journey of these lessons I have collected and start to write a new story for yourself in medicine.

1

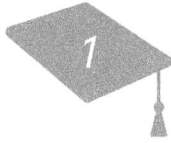

THE MENTORSHIP JOURNEY

I FIRST DECIDED TO SPECIALIZE IN DERMATOLOGY AFTER I realized I enjoyed everything skin-related: I preferred sewing up the leg in cardiac bypass surgery rather than watching the open-heart component for the sixth time, I was excited to discuss the cutaneous drug reactions my assigned patients were experiencing, and I thrived when studying the pediatric patients with neuro-cutaneous syndromes. My dear friend and classmate suggested I consider dermatology as a specialty early in my schooling, but I had no idea there was such a variety of patients. I also didn't realize how competitive the field was. Each time I mentioned my interest to a classmate who was also applying to dermatology, they would ask what my backup plan would be if I didn't match. Even the dean of students asked me that question. I decided early on that I would be *determined* to match rather than come up with an extensive backup plan.

At the time, I didn't have the language or the experience to ask my mentors how to be a great dermatology candidate, let alone consult them on a backup plan. It worked out for me, but the process could have been so much smoother. The bottom line is that finding the right specialty is not enough. You need to have mentorship to plan for the expected *and* the unexpected.

Many students who contact me about dermatology ask me about my story and how I came to the specialty. I usually talk about the clinical things that attracted me to dermatology, but I often fail to mention the mentors who have paved my journey. Mentorship is the backbone of my success in my journey through the many phases of school and my career. I would venture to say that I would never have reached my level of success without others mentoring me—or without the relationships that have been formed through my mentorship of others.

People of color tend to go unnoticed in many fields, with medicine being a primary example, and so they often miss out on these vital mentorship opportunities. One of my goals is to allow those who come behind me to have all the tools possible for success, and I have found that mentorship is the way I can help make this happen. I also find that the more I mentor, the better I get at the job. Each mentoring relationship is a learning experience for me that has carried over into the way I interact with other physicians and with my patients, and even in how I interact with my own children.

Mentoring has become who I am as a person and part of how I define myself. I believe wholeheartedly that the mentorship I have received has to be repaid in kind. Without mentorship, the success of many minoritized high school, college, and medical students is stymied. With mentorship, these students are much more prepared for the curveballs that negative individuals in leadership can throw. For instance, I have witnessed senior physicians ask minoritized students complicated and almost impossible to answer questions rather than actually try to understand the level on which to teach the student. Mentorship can prepare a student for these kinds of experiences and more.

How Does Mentorship Look?

Mentorship can look like many different things. It can be a short conversation about how to structure an application, or it can be a longitudinal experience that lasts for decades. Once I realized that medical students looked up to me when I was just a lowly resident, that lit the fire under me to start mentoring others in a planned and more constructive way. I'd always tried to help those behind me in medical school and residency, but this realization encouraged me to better structure my approach in my mentoring relationships.

I've since made it part of my job to mentor as many students, residents, and early faculty members as possible. I apply for funding to participate in mentoring, I join organizations that value the commitment to mentorship, and I tell my mentees about opportunities to apply for mentorship funds. It is my good luck that the specialty of dermatology has a large tribe of us who are committed to these endeavors. I belong to and actively participate in many organizations that specialize in mentorship, including Women's Dermatologic Society, Skin of Color Society, the American Academy of Dermatology, and the American Hair Research Society.

Mentoring Feedback from Mentor and Mentee Is Key

Most of the learners I mentor are medical students. I especially enjoy mentoring what my psychologist friend calls "emerging adults." Some of my mentees listen to my recommendations and some do not, but that's all part of the process. Some learners I have mentored come back to me years later and tell me how much they appreciated the guidance I shared, and that makes it all worthwhile. Their success is all I need to continue.

> Some of my mentees listen to my recommendations and some do not, but that's all part of the process.

I remember one young applicant to dermatology residency at our medical school. He was a tall, attractive, confident African American medical student. He interviewed moderately well but appeared nervous, so I was willing to chalk up his mediocre answers to nerves and still give him a high ranking for residency since his written application and letters of recommendation were all quite good. I had my ranking ready to go when the administrative assistants who help to set up our residency applicant days overheard this young man trying to ask another residency applicant out on a date while they were waiting to be interviewed by faculty. The other applicant handled his advances in a very professional way, but that unprofessional action was a blemish on this young man's record as far as our faculty were concerned. As a result, he did not get ranked for residency in our program. Unfortunately, he did not match at any other programs that year either.

After not matching, the young man called all the program directors he interviewed with, hoping to get feedback about his performance so he could improve for the next year. I returned his call and was candid about the observation by our administrative assistant as well as his less-than-stellar answers to my interview questions. I also gave several recommendations to strengthen his application for the next cycle. He thanked me and took my recommendations for improvement. After changing his approach and participating in a year of research, he matched into a dermatology program and is now a very successful dermatologist. In fact, every time I see him (and it has been over a decade now), he still thanks me for my honesty and guidance from so many years ago. This young man learned his lesson, and I learned that it helps to tell my students about their behaviors when they are not in line with appropriate professional decorum.

I also learned that many people are not willing to lend a hand to help others up behind them. When I spoke to this young man so many years ago about how to improve his application, he shared with me that not one of the other program directors had returned his call. That's why I do what I do.

> Many people are not willing to lend a hand to help others up behind them.

Mentorship of Fellows

As I moved through my career and research became more important to me, I started to take on a research fellow each year. These fellows are usually either medical students taking a break between their third and fourth years of medical school or physicians who have graduated and completed an internship but haven't yet been able to match into a program. Taking on research fellows is a common practice, and applicants often think of this as a way to secure a position in the competitive specialty of dermatology residency. In many ways this is true, but it is important not to take advantage of these fellows. They are in a precarious position having to work for someone who holds their potential life trajectory in their hands.

When I first began having fellows join me, they were often self-funding their position for the year. I constantly worried about the costs they incurred, but I had no way to fund their work for them. After two of my fellows were able to get funding from their respective medical schools, I began to apply for funding through various mechanisms so that my fellows' financial burdens were not so severe.

But I still think about the fellows at so many other programs who do not have funding. I loathe the idea that we are using these folks for work without giving them what they need to live successfully for that year. Of course, each fellow accepts the unpaid fellowship of their own free will, but the system itself is designed to take advantage of passionate people who just want to get a leg up in the application process for dermatology. I think we all need to take more time to consider how we treat those who are coming behind us and make sure that they have all the necessary support to move forward—whether that be financial help or scholarship opportunities. In the absence of funding, we should embrace purposeful mentoring as a "currency" with which to pay our fellows.

Many of the people that I mentor as research fellows are or were students who were told by their instructors that they were not competitive enough to apply to dermatology or that they were not a good fit. I don't know exactly how all these people found their way to me through referrals and references, but I think they recognize that my claim to fame is helping those who are truly committed to the specialty and who will work hard while enjoying lots of other exposures, including travel for research presentations and interactions with current dermatology residents.

My mentorship during the year of research is 360-degree mentoring, which includes helping the research fellow make contacts with faculty members in our department and outside departments, learn basic dermatology, conduct all parts of research (including writing protocols), and interact with the institutional review board—as well as learn some statistics. They also receive one-on-one mentoring from me, and if they are lucky and smart, they get mentoring from the current residents and other faculty in the department as well.

I have often wished that I had an opportunity to meet and help guide these fellows earlier in their journey in medical school, but I do all that I can at the point that they come to me. It has been a joy to work with these talented young people and see how they grow in maturity and knowledge of the specialty.

My experiences with mentoring have informed my idea of what it takes to be a good mentee. In the best circumstances, all mentees become mentors at some point, and there are some helpful guidelines to consider for mentorship and medicine, particularly as it relates to a competitive specialty.

All mentees become mentors at some point.

For Mentees:

1. Find mentors in those who practice medicine the way you aspire to, even if they are not formal mentors.

2. Listen with an open heart and mind to see what advice rings true and what advice might not work for you.

3. Ask concrete questions of your mentor but make sure to think deeply about them first. You want your questions to be about what you really need rather than ego-stroking questions for your mentor.

4. Decide if a given mentor is to be a short-term or long-term mentor to you, if possible. Consider the interest and time commitment of the mentor. Sometimes the best mentors are those who are only able to mentor for a short time, so you must be open to accepting what they can give and not expect everyone to be a long-term mentor.

5. Tell your mentors when things don't go as planned. Oftentimes, mentees will keep bad news from their mentors because they view it as a failure, but this is an important time to allow your mentor to help you. Honesty is the best policy!

6. Be the one to follow up. Don't expect your mentor to track you down and ask what is happening. Some do and some don't, so check in regularly, perhaps every 4–5 months with an email or a request for a meeting if needed.

This chapter has described what mentorship *can* look like, but mentorship can take many forms. These are just guidelines and my experiences. As we move through the chapters, I will fill in the structure of mentorship with examples and resources.

2

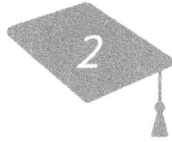

MENTORSHIP AND HOW IT HELPED FORM MY CAREER

THE SUMMER BETWEEN MY FIRST AND SECOND YEAR OF medical school, I was lucky enough to work with a renowned physician and researcher, Dr. Risa Lavizzo-Maury. At that time, she was a clinical and research geriatrician at the University of Pennsylvania Hospital, and importantly, she was a woman of color. She had a quick smile and a great sense of humor. I worked on a small research project with her. Although it didn't lead to any publications, the experience of watching Dr. Lavizzo-Maury on rounds in the nursing home each morning—particularly how she took time to care for these chronically ill, older patients—never left me. She was professional but friendly and always engaged with a smile and questions about their families and important upcoming events. Beyond that, she gave freely of her time to help me focus on my project. She also shared how she approached opportunities in her career and balanced them with her family life.

That summer, Dr. Lavizzo-Maury was living in an undergraduate UPenn dormitory with her family. She was the house mother for a dormitory for African American students, and I thought it was amazing that she would give of herself like this. It impressed me because it was such a departure from anything *my* family would do. I have never forgotten how she described the experience and interwove it with stories about her children. She was a truly gifted person and physician who later became the president and CEO of the Robert Wood Johnson Foundation, the first African American woman to head this organization. She was also named one of the 100 Most Powerful Women by *Forbes* several times. I feel fortunate to have been matched with her as a mentee for a very formative summer, one that has had an enduring impact on my career and life.

Many people have asked me over the years who my early mentors were. Twenty years ago, I would answer that I didn't *have* any early mentors, other than my family members. I didn't know any doctors in my community. No one went to medical school in my family. No one really followed the progression of my career long term until much later in my medical journey, so I considered myself an island when it came to mentors.

But as I reflect on how I made decisions and why I chose certain directions in my life, I realize that I actually did have many mentors, both early in life and throughout my career. We just didn't call them "mentors" back when I was training. The whole area of mentorship was not nearly as well developed as it is now. But considering my time before residency and medical practice, there were certainly people who helped guide my way, albeit some in very small ways.

Formative Year Mentors

Other than my parents and aunts and uncles, my earliest mentor was my first-grade teacher, Miss Starks. She was a strict teacher who seemed to never smile or break the façade of professionalism. She was clear in her expectations—probably a good thing for six-year-olds—and she didn't give an inch when children misbehaved. However, children rarely misbehaved in her class because she had a stern way of looking at you if you seemed like you were about to talk to your neighbor or laugh out of turn. She was a tall, thin woman, dressed impeccably in skirts and blouses or suits. Even her clothes seemed to know how to behave. Her hair was always styled in a neat smooth style, what we might call a curled bob these days. She had smooth, very dark brown skin that seemed to go well with a small streak of gray that ran through her hair.

For me, she was the barometer by which I judged every teacher I had after that. I remember one morning in her class when I was unpacking my book bag. I took out all the books and pencils I would need for the day and realized I hadn't done my homework the night before. I was usually on top of everything with school, and my parents made sure that I stayed that way. I have no idea why I forgot to do my homework that particular night, but sitting right there in my bookbag was the worksheet assignment that I hadn't even started. I was petrified that Miss Starks would view me poorly, but I knew I had to tell her. My desk was in the front of the classroom, so I didn't have far to go to her desk. She must have realized how stressed I was, because when I approached and told her that I had forgotten to do the assignment, her usual stern face softened, and she said that it was fine to complete the assignment that evening and turn it in the next day. She never mentioned it again, but I never forgot that kindness. She showed me how a no-nonsense approach can work—but you have to show some mercy when it's called for.

> A no-nonsense approach can work—but you have to show some mercy when it's called for.

Interestingly, I recently read a study in the book *Hidden Potential* by Adam Grant showing that the experience of a child's kindergarten teacher can determine their later character.[1] It influences how proactive, pro-social, disciplined, and determined children are later in life. Now it makes perfect sense that my early teacher was such a memorable person to me. She was a big part of strengthening my character and self-identity.

Miss Starks never married or had children, but she certainly knew what she was doing with all of us kids. My sister had had Miss Starks as her first-grade teacher five years before, so we knew she was an excellent teacher, and we both felt a sense of mentorship from her. Every year after, Miss Starks sent us each a card on our birthdays, and we wrote one back to her for her birthday. This practice lasted into our adulthood. Miss Starks and I shared a birthday, and I always looked forward to seeing her card each year, as she usually wrote an encouraging sentence or two in the card. I received the last card from her sometime during my residency, and my sister and I assumed that she had passed away as my sister stopped receiving cards at that time as well. We never knew if she wrote them to all her students or just the ones who showed promise, or maybe she continued sending us cards because we also sent her cards back. Whatever the reason, our year with her at a very impressionable time and her follow up with me and my sister showed me that mentors can show up in your life as scary or unlikely characters. It's up to you to recognize them by their actions.

High School Mentor

As I made my way through school, I met several people whom I now consider mentors. One was a high school English teacher, Teacher Janet (in Quaker schools we used the Quaker way of addressing teachers: the word "teacher" and their first name). Teacher Janet was another one of those exacting teachers who ran a tight ship—again something needed with rowdy teenagers. She was able to quiet a class just by raising her hand slightly and looking at all the students slowly. I never heard her raise her voice or say a negative thing to a student, but she was also a bit unapproachable because of her stoic and straight-faced manner. I loved her classes because she really knew literature and had the most interesting prompts for our writing assignments. She inspired her students to be creative with their writing and truly seemed to enjoy reading students' papers.

In my junior year of high school, after she had graded several of my assignments, Teacher Janet asked me to come to her classroom for a meeting during my free period. She was so deadpan and dour when she said it, I thought for sure I was in some kind of trouble. When I went to see her, she asked me to sit and told me that my writing was excellent and that I had a gift. She encouraged me to submit something to the school magazine, which I did. The magazine published my piece, and I was quite proud of that achievement. No one else seemed overly impressed with my writing, but I'll never forget the feeling of someone telling me I was doing something well and that I should push to do more.

Dermatology Residency Mentor

Another time I didn't realize I was being mentored was during my dermatology residency. I was in my third and final year and was starting to consider work options after residency. I was dating a young man who was a Michigan resident, so I was contemplating jobs there but also felt the pull to return home to Philadelphia. I also had to study for board exams and complete my regular workload. I even had a moonlighting job on Saturdays in Detroit, driving just over an hour to and from a clinic where I worked to make extra money. I was feeling a bit overwhelmed with it all and certainly was not interested in entertaining more work.

However, that was exactly what one of my faculty members asked me to do. He asked me to start working on a clinical study that looked at using a retinoid cream to help prevent detrimental thinning of the skin with topical steroid use. The research was interesting, but when the project was over, he asked me to write the paper to publish our results. I had never written a scientific paper, and I just couldn't see it as anything other than more work on top of all I was already doing. Many years later, I realized that my faculty member had been exposing me to clinical research and publishing in an academic journal, which is a valuable lesson to learn! I did finally stop dragging my feet on the project and attempted to write the paper. Many drafts later (and red-pen markups on his part), the article was published in a major dermatology journal.

After that, I was bitten by the research bug and was forever grateful to the faculty member for seeing something in me that I certainly didn't. Sometimes the extra work pushes you to a new level. There is no question that he could have written that article in his sleep in less time than it took me to write the title and the abstract. But he allowed me to struggle through five or six rough drafts and was patient and thoughtful as he taught me. The lesson here is to recognize that sometimes work is just work, but sometimes extra work can be a gift that you need to accept gracefully, as it will push you to the next step in your career.

> Sometimes work is just work, but sometimes extra work can be a gift.

I'd be remiss if I didn't mention the doctor I worked for in my moonlighting job. Again, I was living my life and didn't consider him to be a mentor. His name was Dr. Robert Heidelberg, and he was the owner of a large private practice in Detroit, Michigan, serving primarily African American patients. At that time, he owned one of the very few practices that catered to this population in Detroit. His patient numbers were ridiculously high, so he always needed help despite working Monday through Friday, evenings on Tuesday, and Saturday mornings. The University of Michigan residents had a tradition of moonlighting in the offices of private practice dermatologists; it was a win-win situation where the residents could all make extra money and the private office could see more patients.

That was how this job was presented to me by an upper-level resident who was graduating from the program. Specifically, the upper-level resident told me that there was a Black doctor in Detroit who always employed Black residents from the University of Michigan and the Henry Ford Hospital Durham residency programs. None of the other local offices had ever extended a moonlighting job to Black residents, so Dr. Heidelberg was the one opportunity I had for moonlighting. I eagerly pursued my full license to practice in Michigan after my second year out of med school and joined Dr. Heidelberg every Saturday morning in Detroit to see patients. Dr Heidelberg was a tall, attractive, older Black man with a ready smile and kind eyes. He had a very calm and pleasant manner and never really directed our treatment as moonlighters. He did have certain regimens that he followed, so his nurses taught us how to follow these guidelines when seeing patients in his office.

In his clinic, we needed three kinds of intralesional corticosteroid injections: low concentration for injecting acne lesions, middle concentration for alopecia, and high concentration for keloids. We did a similar thing in our academic clinics, but it was never as clear or succinct as it was in Dr. Heidelberg's office because our academic practices were not monolithic in terms of the race of patients. From Dr. Heidelberg, I learned about the conditions seen in patients of African American descent.

What an education I received at the clinic over two years of Saturday mornings! Dr. Heidelberg's daughter now runs his practice, and thank goodness there are now more Black dermatologists in Detroit than when I was working there. This experience was informal mentoring, which is a helpful experience at all levels of medical training. His informal mentorship helped me realize that I wanted to do clinical practice but not just by seeing clinical patients. I learned that I wanted to specialize in patients with skin of color because so many of the common conditions seen were not well studied nor were there well-worked-out treatment regimens.

This helped me make the decision to include clinical research in my future career as a dermatologist.

Mentors After Entering Academic Medicine

Once I reached my academic home at Wake Forest School of Medicine, I had lots of mentors. One of the most important in my career was the founding chair of the department, Dr. Joe Jorizzo. He was the match that ignited a fire in all the clinical faculty in the department and made the place an amazing incubator of clinical expertise and clinical research excellence. But there was another person who had a profound effect on me, even though she was only in our department for a short time.

Dr. Gloria Graham was a legend in dermatology. She was called the mother of liquid nitrogen because she had described so many ways that the substance could be used in clinical dermatology, many of which are still in use. She lived in or around North Carolina but had always practiced in private practice. She had attended Wake Forest School of Medicine as one of the first few women to be admitted into the medical school back when the school was called Bowman Gray School of Medicine. She kept connections with the medical school alumni office and alerted them that she was moving back to the Winston Salem area with her husband, who had recently retired from his career as a dermatopathologist. The chair of our department got wind of her return and approached her about working part time in our department. Dr. Graham had recently recovered from Guillain-Barré syndrome, a condition that causes severe muscle weakness due to an inflammatory attack on peripheral nerves. As a result, she didn't want to work full time and thought the job in our department would be a nice way to wind her career down. It did not turn out to be a good "wind-down" job since we were a bustling young department with lots of needs, so Gloria did not stay for very long.

Gloria *did* stay long enough for me to see and learn about grace. I am not a graceful person, and no one in my family is particularly graceful—literally or figuratively—so this was not something I knew much about. Gloria had grace in spades. She was just a lovely person who treated everyone as a new and exciting prospective friend. She never rushed anyone through a story, and she truly listened when you talked to her.

She was particularly kind to me and my daughter, inviting us to a ballet with her. It was my daughter's first time seeing a ballet. My husband got her all dressed up in her finest dress and shoes for the event so that Gloria and I could leave directly from work. It was a lovely night, one my daughter, who was four years old at the time, still remembers.

Sometimes when I'm in a room with a patient, I remember the grace that Gloria showed everyone she met, and it makes me slow down to really listen and give counsel that shows grace. I may come out of the patient room and grumble about not being able to stay on time, which isn't very graceful, but I'm a much better doctor because of Gloria's example. Sometimes it's not what mentors *tell* you or what you read about. Sometimes, the best lessons come from simply paying attention to those around you and watching how they approach the world.

Sometimes, the best lessons come from simply paying attention to those around you and watching how they approach the world.

We can all learn to have more grace, especially in current times when this seems to be a forgotten trait. As I stated, grace does not come to me naturally, so I have to take stock of my behavior when I get rushed or have a particularly difficult day. That's when I am least likely to show grace. Having Gloria model this for me was a great mentoring gift. In some ways I am following her lead, as she also wrote a book about mentoring, but her book was for our fellow colleagues to highlight mentors and mentorship in dermatology. Unfortunately, Gloria passed away recently, so she won't get the chance to read this book, but her spirit lives on in so many of us for whom she modeled grace in medicine and in life.

Recommendations on Picking Your Mentors

Mentorship is now a popular concept. There are set mentors for medical students as they enter school. These assigned mentors are often trained to help students navigate the ups and downs of school. However, sometimes they aren't a great match for students or don't have the information that the student needs to be successful.

Take advantage of *any* mentor you're assigned. Often, students won't seek the help of an assigned mentor because they fear they won't be helpful or that they won't understand them culturally. Get over these potentially untrue beliefs! If you find that the assigned mentor is not able to cover all that you need, it is perfectly fine to seek the advice of others in leadership for a possible mentorship relationship. There are various organizations in the specialty of dermatology that offer mentorship

Take advantage of *any* mentor you're assigned.

grants for students and residents. These opportunities will often pay for the experience and even give a stipend.

Also, be aware that if you've chosen someone as a mentor and they are not a willing participant, the mentorship is not likely to move forward, so be open to moving on if someone is a great leader but not the best mentor. There may be other ways you can work with that leader besides mentorship.

Finally, examine those around you who model the behaviors that you'd like to have or that you admire. Recognize that they may be undercover mentors for you. Also, recognize that you can learn from the opportunities that you're offered, so make sure to take advantage of opportunities that may seem like work, as they may be the most fruitful experiences that you have.

If there doesn't seem to be a mentor in dermatology with whom you can work, consider a physician in another specialty who seems open to teaching and has a reputation for treating students well. Often, this can be a longitudinal relationship, with their connections helping you to pursue your interests.

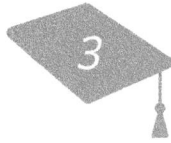

3

BELONGING

How Can I Feel at Home in Medicine?

FEELING LIKE YOU DON'T BELONG—ESPECIALLY IF YOU'RE Black—can diminish your promotion in medicine on an individual basis, but it doesn't have to change the spark of genius that helps patients. This is the story of Dr. Percy Lavon Julian.

Dr. Julian was a Black biochemist who revolutionized the synthesis of corticosteroids. He was the grandson of a slave, and even though he was forced to live in off-campus housing that refused to serve him meals, he achieved Phi Beta Kappa at his undergraduate school. He went on to Harvard for his master's degree but was not able to complete his PhD because the white students would not accept a Black instructor. He was turned away from many jobs because of his race but finally completed his degree in Europe and found a job at a US company where, in 1949, he discovered how to synthesize corticosteroids on a massive scale from soybeans.

Despite his work success and the fact that he ultimately changed the face of medicine with his discoveries, his home was bombed and he was the victim of arson. His story shows us that *belonging* does not go hand in hand with an advanced degree or success in your medical pursuits. It also shows that *not* belonging shouldn't hold you back from achieving your career goals.

In dermatology, we have our own pioneer. His name was Dr. John Kenney, MD. He was one of the first Black dermatologists, the first Black dermatology chairperson, the first Black resident at the University of Michigan Department of Dermatology, and the first Black member of the American Academy of Dermatology Board of Directors. He was also the first to study and elevate "ethnic skin" as a topic for academic research. Similar to Dr. Julian, Dr. Kenney's family was terrorized because of their race, but this didn't keep him from greatly advancing the science of ethnic skin in dermatology. As a result of his experiences, Dr. Kenney started a legacy that helped those of color feel that they belong as patients and providers in the field of dermatology.

Belonging in Current Times

Why am I telling you these stories? Because others have already laid the groundwork for the rest of us (so we don't have it nearly as hard as they did), and because we still need to improve how people of color are treated in medicine—separate from our scientific studies and successes. We must understand our past if we are to be successful in the future.

We must understand our past if we are to be successful in the future.

It is easy to be happy that you've found a good mentor, performed research in dermatology, or maybe even published and presented at meetings. These are all amazing milestones in your medical career. But they don't directly contribute to ensuring those coming behind you are accepted and feel that they belong. We must still work in the area of "belonging" and give back.

Belonging is now studied as part of the science of discrimination. You can think of belonging as a psychological safety in your environment. When you feel psychologically safe, you feel you'll be given the benefit of the doubt. You ask questions and raise issues without fear of retribution. This allows for high-performing teams, where members build and learn and grow together, push back against the status quo, and innovate.[2] Verna Meyers, a Netflix VP of Inclusion, stated, "Diversity is being invited to the party, Inclusion is being asked to dance . . . and Belonging is knowing all the songs."[3]

The summary definition of belonging is *being seen, connected, supported, and proud*. Each of these can be an issue for patients as well as providers. Patients of color may not feel that their cultural behaviors are understood. This is particularly true of haircare practices and those who see the dermatologist for hair loss. Many patients are referred to me because an outside dermatologist voiced incomplete knowledge of haircare practices and hair loss for the people of color. We know that by the year 2050, the US will be a majority-minority country, so most dermatologists will need to understand how to approach skin-of-color patients—and all the cultural behaviors that come with them.

Belonging is being seen, connected, supported, and proud.

It would not be acceptable for me to tell a white patient that I don't know anything about skin cancer or cultural behaviors that might contribute to its development. To visually reveal this dichotomy, I like to show the photography of the artist Endia Beal, who has an amazing exhibition called "Can I Touch It." Her work shows white women in work suits with culturally typical hairstyles of Black women such as cornrows, box braids, and short afros, showing that hair is just hair—and that there is no reason dermatologists shouldn't be knowledgeable about all kinds of hair and cultural haircare practices. Patients will be more comfortable if they have culturally competent providers, allowing them to feel they belong when they come to the doctor.

How Can You Feel Like You Belong

Belonging is a process that may start with getting together with other BIPOC (Black, indigenous, and people of color) students, particularly those who are ahead of you in medical school. It may mean taking advantage of the Student National Medical Association (I will describe this more later) at your school, or it may mean that *you* must help build a community.

Another organization that helps URiM (underrepresented in medicine) students who seek to become dermatologists is Nth Dimensions. Nth Dimensions was founded in 2004 by Dr. Bonnie Simpson-Mason, an orthopedic surgeon. She initially helped students interested in orthopedic surgery but then started working with the American Academy of Dermatology (AAD) to help dermatology residency applicants in 2018. Dr. Henry Lim was the President of the AAD at the time, and a big focus of his presidency was focus on racial equity in dermatology. This program mentors medical students throughout medical school until graduation with in-person sessions, faculty mentors, and summer experiences, all geared toward improving chances of matching in their respective specialty of dermatology or orthopedic surgery.

If there are no prominent organizations at your medical school, finding others interested in diversity can be a start. There are usually interested people in these environments who will help you feel you are an important part of the community. Finding outside organizations, such as the National Medical Association, dermatology section, or the Skin of Color Society, and working on committees with these groups will give you a sense of belonging while you also help push the field of diversity forward.

How Can You Contribute to Others' Feeling of Belonging

Medical students of color can contribute to others' feeling of belonging while seeing patients on rotation by making sure patients' concerns are heard and understood. That might mean spending a few more minutes with the patient after the outpatient visit, as long as the faculty member agrees. Patients enjoy added special education, and students can make them feel that sense of belonging.

Students can also help by volunteering at clinics for underserved populations to increase patient access to care. If your medical school does not have such a clinic, you can get permission to start one. If you see a patient need that isn't being addressed at a free clinic, perhaps you and other students can brainstorm options for them. This is a win-win for patients and allows you to show your leadership potential. These ideas do not have to be dermatology-related, so don't worry about that. *Any* innovation that helps patients would be great. These approaches help you build a more well-rounded application, and you will also feel useful while helping these patients feel a sense of belonging.

Dermatology Applicant Diversity and Belonging

I will share just a bit of the wealth of available data about dermatology applicant belonging. The diversity within dermatology doesn't reflect the US population. In fact, Black dermatologists in the US are approximately 4% of the total, while the US population prevalence of those who self-identify as Black is estimated at 12.1%, according to the US Census.[4] According to AAMC data, during the 2023–2024 academic year, the national percentage of Black or African American males applying to medical school was 2.7%, while only 2.9% matriculated—a number that has remained relatively stagnant since 1978 despite an overall increase in the number of Black male college graduates.[5] These circumstances are key in understanding why people of color don't feel like they belong in dermatology.

A study was performed of dermatology applicants at one department for the 2018–2019 cycle, examining racial breakdown and various factors of interest for applicants.[6] In this study, 149 and 142 dermatology applicants completed initial 2019 and 2020 surveys, respectively, then 112 and 124 completed the follow-up surveys. The racial breakdown was 69.9% Caucasian, 23.7% Asian, 5.4% African American, 0.4% American Indian/Alaska Native, and 0.7% Native Hawaiian/Pacific Islander; 8% identified as Hispanic/Latino. URiM applicants published more papers and took our more educational loans than white or Asian applicants. URiM applicants also completed more pre-residency research fellowships compared to white applicants. Despite all of this, URiM applicants were less likely to match (76.7%) vs. white (88.4%) and Asian (96.0%; p=0.03). The median Step 1 scores were lower for underrepresented applicants in medicine URiM (p<0.01), but of course this is no longer a factor since Step 1 is now pass/fail. There were no observed differences in away rotations or interviews attended. (This suggests that comparable experience and scores do not even the playing field for URiM students in the competitive match for dermatology.)

The good news is that there are many program directors and chairs of departments, not to mention CEOs and deans of medical schools, who recognize that diversity in medicine is absolutely essential to care for all populations in the United States. Many published papers have enumerated recommendations for how to increase diversity in dermatologic residencies, including the following:

- Making diversity an explicit goal of residency selection
- Shifting emphasis from test scores and publication numbers, valuing other applicant qualities based on quality, not quantity (e.g., leadership, teamwork, teaching skills, innovative vision, commitment to underserved)
- Changing the residency interview format (virtual interviews may work best for URiM applicants who may not have funding for extensive travel for in-person interviews)
- Prioritizing other competencies in addition to medical knowledge

- Recruiting and retaining more URiM academic physicians as mentors

This means that applicants of color need to include other qualities in their applications, even if it may not seem important. The Association of American Medical Colleges recommends a holistic review of medical school applicants involving a balanced consideration of experiences, attributes, and academic metrics. These metrics are slowly being adopted in dermatology departments. For example, distance traveled (from single parent family, first generation American, URiM, self-financed education, etc.) is important to describe if applicable (and if you're comfortable sharing).

> Applicants of color need to include other qualities in their applications, even if it may not seem important.

Right now, diversity and equity are controversial topics. As time goes on, this may change, and it may not always be important for every residency applicant committee to hear about your status as a URiM or issues that only affect patients of color (see more about this in the section on the Personal Statement). You can start thinking about this early in your medical school career, no matter what specialty of medicine you plan on. Other important achievements might include the commitment of the applicant to address healthcare disparities, leadership, volunteerism, excellence in sports, and other life experiences.

To feel a sense of belonging, it is important to remember the past, as it has helped many of us to achieve success in our specialty. Data supports the current lack of diversity in the field and demonstrates that patients prefer race-concordant visits and better outcomes have been reported as well. Each of us can help in achieving belonging for patients, students, and practicing physicians.

Microaggressions in Medicine and How to Handle Them

During medical school, whenever a microaggression occurred, I just adopted a "here we go again" mentality. One of those times, I was on the neurology service and all the residents, students, and attending on the team were white men. On the first day of the rotation, everyone on the team introduced themselves and told where they went to college. I would have been the last one, but when my turn came, the attending physician simply told me to go get the patient charts instead of allowing me to report my college. As it happened, my undergraduate college was much more highly ranked than anyone else's, not that it mattered to me. I simply gave myself a silent peptalk because I was not going to let this microaggression make me think less of myself. But there are better ways to recognize and address these situations.

Starting a conversation about microaggression may not seem necessary unless someone has just said something to you that was egregious or discriminatory, but the time to talk about this is *not* when you are in the midst of a racially charged or biased situation. Instead, you need time to reflect and gain perspective on how to handle these situations when they arise. It may seem strange to consider *preparing* for a bad or biased situation, almost like you are looking for trouble,

> You need time to reflect and gain perspective on how to handle these situations when they arise.

but it's just the opposite. If you can spot trouble coming down the road, you can avoid getting in the way and help avert the danger it presents.

What Are Microaggressions?

The term "racial microaggression" was first coined in 1970 by Professor Chester Pierce. Microaggressions are described as brief and commonplace daily verbal, behavioral, and environmental indignities, whether *intentional* or *unintentional*, that communicate hostile, derogatory, or negative racial, gender, sexual orientation, social class, or religious slights and insults to the target person or group.

I want to discuss this topic for URiM students, particularly those who want to apply to competitive residencies, because not knowing how to handle microaggressions can cost you grades, evaluations, and research opportunities. Examples in medicine include demeaning comments, nonverbal disrespect, generalizations of social identity, assumption of nonphysician status, role—or credential-questioning behavior, explicit epithets, rejection of care, questioning or inquiries of ethnic/racial origin, and sexual harassment.

Not knowing how to handle microaggressions can cost you grades, evaluations, and research opportunities.

When I was in medical school, none of these behaviors were labeled. No one knew about microaggressions as a term, and when these things happened, my URiM friends and I just sucked it up or talked about it among ourselves. As more focus has been placed on racial equity recently, it's imperative to recognize when these behaviors are directed at you and how to respond appropriately.

While in my residency, I encountered an elderly white man who refused to allow me to examine him in the dermatology clinic because he felt that I was only in my position due to affirmative action. This patient's words shook me to my core. When I reported what happened to my supervising faculty member, he just said not to worry about it and to move onto the next patient. This was *not* the way to handle a microaggression or to support someone at whom the microaggression was directed. I was unable to concentrate on work for the rest of the day. It was an awful encounter, forever etched in my memory. That kind of experience makes you less effective as a learner, takes up space in your brain, and can disconnect you from the work of learning and caring for patients.

Types of Microaggression

Implicit bias is a form of interpersonal racism, and microaggressions represent a specific form of implicit bias. Those who commit microaggressions may see them as misunderstandings of intent (an innocent question or simple mistake); for example, telling an African American they are a credit to their race or asking brown people where they are from and not accepting their first answer when it is not a foreign country. These are hurtful experiences that prevent URiM learners from focusing on the act of learning medicine because they impose the burden of extra cognitive work to deal with them. If you understand the different types of microaggressions, you have a better chance of responding and moving past them.

There are four major types that have been described.

1. The first is **microassault**, which involves explicit and intentional discriminatory actions by verbal or nonverbal attacks against someone's identity with intention to hurt the victim through name calling, avoidant behavior, or purposeful discriminatory actions.

2. The second type is **microinsult**, characterized by nonverbal or verbal remarks or comments that convey rudeness and insensitivity that demean a person's heritage or identity.

3. The third type is **microinvalidations**, which are verbal comments or behaviors that exclude, negate, or nullify the thoughts, feelings, or experiential reality of a person's identity.

4. The fourth type is **environmental** and occurs when URiMs do not see themselves represented in course, books, theories or are not presented with materials that showcase a non-majority perspective.

I recommend reading the book by Damon Tweedy called *Black Man in a White Coat: A Doctor's Reflections on Race and Medicine*.[7] The author is a psychiatrist who attended medical school and residency at Duke University in North Carolina. He reflects on his experience as a medical student when a professor mistakenly assumed he was a maintenance worker in the classroom. Tweedy describes how he internalized the exchange and, despite his success throughout the course of his medical training, combatted feelings of anxiety, self-doubt, and implied inferiority. While he doesn't speak in terms of microaggressions, this situation hit both the microinsult and microinvalidation types.

At the end of the day, it is important for minoritized people to know that they are not alone when they feel singled out by a microaggression. The knowledge that there are specific and recognizable forms of microaggression helps take a bit of the emotional sting out of the experience—and may help you prepare to respond.

Responding to Microaggressions

Less than a decade ago, a first-year medical student at my school wanted to initiate survey questions to her fellow classmates about microaggressions. She went through the appropriate process to get the questions approved for the typical survey distributed to the first-year class after every set of exams. Everything seemed to be in order until several faculty members became concerned that the questions would offend white students.

This student was directed to me because I perform racial equity research. I had a psychologist friend who studies microaggressions with a focus on young Black women, so I introduced the two. My friend helped the student develop her argument that the questions should be included—and ultimately, they were added to the class survey. This student was able to collect the data and present a poster at a national meeting. She saw a problem, figured out how to investigate the issue, and stayed on task even in the face of challenge. She's something of a phenom anyway, completing an MD/PhD and going on to a vascular surgery residency, and she exemplifies the way to respond to microaggressions—with investigation and interest in improving the situation.

Currently, most medical centers have groups for reporting observed microaggressions.[8] They have slogans and processes in place for identifying and addressing all types of discrimination in the medical environment. This is one outcome of the focus on violence against underrepresented minorities during the pandemic. However, there is always work to do; not everyone is at the same place on the racial equity journey.

I find it difficult to be ready for a biased comment in the moment. When I have experienced them, I am often focused on something so completely different that I am caught off guard. The comments may come from patients, a colleague, or someone in a leadership position. One recent microaggression toward me was clearly unintentional and from a typically supportive person in a leadership position. I was undergoing treatment for a serious and somewhat rare medical condition. When I discussed it with this leader, they asked me if this condition occurred in Black people. Clearly, I was a Black person with the condition, but I considered the source of the comment and did not speak up at that time.

Thinking about this now, it might have been best to gently correct this leader. Even those of us who are aware of these strategies must constantly work on using them. Generally, I think of the best comeback long after the interaction has passed, but there are several frameworks to consider in real-time with someone saying or doing something that feels like a microaggression.

First, it is imperative to determine if a response is appropriate, safe, and likely to be helpful in each individual situation. Then, you can choose the appropriate framework. All the frameworks I discuss

Determine if a response is appropriate, safe, and likely to be helpful in each individual situation.

have been worked out by others (see references). One framework is ACTION.[9]

1. "A" stands for **Asking clarifying questions** like "I want to make sure I understood what you said. What did you mean when you said _____?".

2. You need to **Come from a place of Curiosity** ("C"), not judgment. Listen intently to how they explain their statement and give them space to clarify.

3. Then you can **Tell** ("T") them what you observed in a factual way. "What I heard you say was . . . ."

4. The next letter, "I," stands for **Impact Exploration**, where you can ask how they think this comment can impact or be perceived by certain groups.

5. "O" is for **Own your own thoughts and feelings** about the impact. "Many people might take that comment to mean _____."

6. Finally, "N" is for **Next Steps**. Request appropriate action be taken. You can ask the commenter to refrain from making comments like this because it offends members of the group and does not allow them to focus.

Another approach would be to use the XYZ technique: "I feel X when you say Y because Z." If neither of these feels right for you, you can consider the "Open the Front Door" method: Observe, Think, Feel, Desire. Perhaps this framework would have been good to share with the leader in my case. I could have said, "Your question is interesting since I am a Black person [observe]. I think that this condition does not know my color [think], and I feel that disease does not respect race or ethnicity [feel]. My hope is that we all can remember this as we treat patients [desire]."

There are more frameworks out there as well, including the ERASE framework: Expect, Recognize, Address, Support, and Encourage.[10] Described by Goldenberg et al., the overall concept is like the rest. You must expect that microaggressions will happen so you aren't caught off guard. That means you must *practice* what you will say prior to when the bias occurs. Then you must *recognize* the type of microaggression that is occurring and determine if and how to address the issue.

> Be the impetus for positive cultural change in your community.

We haven't discussed the necessary environmental support, but that's also critically important. Not only do you need to be supportive of others to whom this happens, but you also need to be the impetus for positive cultural change in your community.

How to Minimize Likelihood of Microaggressions in Your Environment

Intervention strategies to reduce the likelihood of the occurrence of microaggressions should include cultivating allies, followed by demanding accountability in your immediate environment.[11] Allies are members of the majority group who collectively collaborate with members of the non-majority group to effect change through promoting diversity, equity, and inclusion.

Cultivating allies involves building a network of collaboration that emphasizes education. Education is critical for allies to address microaggressions at the interpersonal level. This process of education involves self-reflection and self-awareness in exploring your biases, fears, and assumptions. We all have biases, and you will be best able to move the needle in this area if you have looked inward first. You might have some difficult or uncomfortable conversations. Educate others about microaggressions—don't just awkwardly laugh and cringe on the outside. Be an ALLY! Tell them why they are wrong!

You can use your mentors and colleagues to help you navigate microaggressions as well. Discussing the experiences can help diffuse anger, fear, and sadness and help you see how to better handle similar situations in the future.

> Educate others about microaggressions. Be an ALLY!

Demanding structural accountability means that you try to work at reducing microaggression at the larger systemic level. This strategy involves implicit bias and antiracism training and the identification of mentors who can help. This is your chance to be a leader and make sure your future is secure—while also building a legacy for improving the lives of others.

4

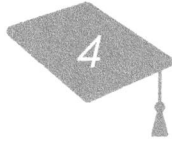

How Early Challenges Can Color Your Career in Medicine

I INCLUDE THIS CHAPTER BECAUSE IT'S IMPORTANT FOR young learners to recognize that all skin-of-color leaders in dermatology have had to experience and weather microaggressions during their lifetime. Some are egregious and others are minor, but all take a toll on the body, the mind, and the focus you have during your career. Here, I share just a couple of these early experiences to show that you *can* get through them—and that you can move forward without the negative feelings they often engender. You don't forget them, but you can utilize them to inform your decisions on handling future microaggressions.

The Cost of Microaggression

The summer before I was to begin college at Swarthmore College, I became short-tempered with my family, grouchy, and just an overall mean person. None of this was typical of my personality or behavior, and thank goodness my mother recognized that something was wrong. She came into my room one evening after a particularly snide comment I made. She gently sat on the side of my twin bed, the one I had slept on for my entire life, and asked what was going on. It was then that I realized I was stressed because I thought I wasn't smart enough to go to Swarthmore.

At first, it was very nice that everyone talked about what a great school Swarthmore was and how well they prepared their students. But the more great things people said, the more I felt like I must have been admitted to the school by mistake and that I would be a failure. My mother gave me a brief pep talk about her and my dad's support—and the fact that I was just as smart as the other students and would do great at college. She was a woman of few words, so this talk was succinct and to the point . . . just what I needed. I figured she knew me better than anyone, and she was one of the smartest people I knew. I dropped the fear and got back to my usual calm demeanor.

Once I arrived at Swarthmore later that summer, I felt the excitement to meet new friends, awe at the beauty of the campus (an arboretum with the most amazing plants and trees), and determination to make my family proud. There was *no* fear.

I had two roommates: a lacrosse player from New Hampshire and a loud math major from Connecticut. Within hours of meeting them, the math major told me I should've sent my photo into the freshman information book, something I hadn't felt the need to do. It became quite clear that she wished I'd sent my photo in because she didn't want to live with a Black person.

Several weeks into the semester, the math major told me a long story about her best friend who didn't get into the college of her choice because a Black student from their high school was admitted with inferior grades and less impressive activities. I suggested that no one other than the admissions committee could possibly know how the applications compared—and that hundreds of students were admitted, so how could anyone know the truth? My loud roommate insisted that *she* knew, and that was that. So it began: the bias, the discrimination that so often creeps in when people are set believing in the inferiority of people of color. It may take weeks or months in a new environment, but in my experience, it's always there, lurking, ready to interfere.

I largely ignored the clearly prejudiced roommate. My other roommate was an incredibly bright and kind person who, interestingly, spent time with our loud, unkind roommate. When I asked her why, she said that although *I* had quickly found friends among the Black students on campus and the other lacrosse players were there for *her*, the loud woman—surprise—had not made many friends. I appreciated her altruism, but it wasn't lost on me that she was supporting someone who was actively biased against a full segment of society while incapable of finding her own group in college.

Life went on that semester. I just didn't think often of my prejudiced roommate, until one day I saw her walking toward me as I was coming from class to exchange my books. It was a beautiful fall day, and campus was crowded with students. All was well with the world until I saw that she was wearing *my* shirt! She hadn't asked me if she could wear my clothes; we hadn't discussed sharing anything in our room. When I approached and questioned her about it, she said I had so many clothes that she didn't think it mattered and that I could wear her clothes if I wanted. I politely informed her that I didn't have any interest in wearing her clothes and that I bought my clothes with money from all the jobs I'd had since age fourteen, including while in college.

She laughed and said I was very stingy. The next week, she made a big deal about buying me a gift. It was a notebook, for which I thanked her. Then I saw the cover photo on the notebook was of Miss Piggy (the dressy pig from the Muppets). Nevertheless, I told her I absolutely loved it, and I used that notebook every day for the rest of the semester. Her juvenile actions were no match for the kind of racial violence I had witnessed, discussed, and avoided for my entire life in Philadelphia, but it still took energy and a small part of my brain to respond to her pokes at me.

People who haven't experienced discrimination don't realize that it's like a movie playing in the back of your mind. You may be having a good time with friends, enjoying a spring day, or dancing at a party, but the movie is always playing at a low level, getting louder whenever a discriminatory act occurs. It can become the main feature when the discrimination is particularly violent or egregious. The schoolgirl shenanigans of my roommate did not rate highly, and as such, the movie stayed at a low level. But it takes energy to keep this movie playing as a warning mechanism and can lead to stress.

Perhaps it was easy for me to simply move past the roommate issues because they were not standing in the way of anything important. I recognized early on that she would not be a friend—just the opposite. She was a prejudiced elitist who used microaggressions to assuage her own feeling of inadequacy and jealousy. It was *not* as easy to write off the bias from a person of power at the college, someone who could change the trajectory of my educational experience.

Putting Past Microaggressions from Superiors into Perspective

In the fall semester of my junior year at college, a new professor came to campus to start a computer science major. He was introduced at a student event one evening where he gave a presentation about his course offerings. This was 1984, and computer science was just burgeoning. In my small private high school, we'd had exactly two computers available to students, and I never needed to use them. This was also a time when floppy disks ruled. The new professor gave an inspiring speech about the classes he would be teaching and how they could benefit any student, no matter their main course of study. He looked trustworthy with his comfortable college professor uniform of khaki pants and a V-neck sweater. He was a bit fatherly with his well-trimmed salt-and-pepper beard.

I did my due diligence to make sure this class could work for me. I asked my pre-med counselor if I could take the course pass/fail. She stated that under no circumstances should a pre-med student take a course pass/fail because it made the student look lazy and would make my transcript less desirable. I went to meet with the computer science professor and discussed my heavy load of science courses for my biology major and my concern that this was so foreign that it could take more time than I could spare. He assured me that I'd be fine in the introductory class and would have no problems keeping up.

Fast forward to me in the class. On the first day, the professor stated that eight out of ten points would be given for the homework assignments, and the extra two points could only be earned if something extra was added to the program. This did not sound fair to me and was nothing like the usually very fair grading practices of other courses at my college. But I pushed on. Very quickly, it was clear that most of the students in the class were quite familiar with computer science programming; most were freshmen and had experience in high school. Just two years had made a big difference in the knowledge base of these younger students, most of whom took the class only as a requirement for the upper-level classes.

For some reason, I just could not get the hang of computer programming, so I sought out a free tutor. The tutor helped me understand the idea of the "loop" and "if/then" statements that were a backbone of programming. He taught me the basic dogma of computer science, the things I wasn't grasping from class or the textbook, and I happily sent him on his way after a couple of weeks. I was still spending hours completing the homework (to the detriment of my other work), but I now understood the basics of programming.

However, I bombed the first test. I was used to tests that assessed a deep understanding of the material, but this test required memorization of at least five kinds of programs that had to be written out during the one-hour test. I needed to configure these programs from my memory of the basic premises, and I simply ran out of time and failed the test. For the second test, I memorized as much as I could while trying to balance all my other work. When I only did marginally better on the second test, I went to speak with the professor about the test to try to figure out this different way of studying.

Before I could finish my explanation, he accused me of cheating. He said that no one who could do so well on homework assignments should have done so poorly on the tests. He knew that I had used a tutor and suggested that they were doing my homework for me. I explained that I did not cheat, period. Not in his class and not in any way in my life, as this was not the ethic I learned in my home or in my Quaker school, nor was it doctrine at Swarthmore. This college was about improving yourself by inquiry and finding your own interests and strengths through education.

Perhaps because I was pre-med and concerned about grades, he didn't believe a word I was saying. It was clear I could not budge his assumptions about me, so I asked a vice dean of students to act as an intermediary in a discussion with the professor. During this second conversation, he allowed one concession—I could pass the course if I did well on the final. Otherwise, he would fail me for cheating.

When final time came, the finals for all my other classes were on the first two days of the week, and my computer science final was five days later, allowing me the time to memorize the entire textbook for the class. This truly seemed like a gift from God. My goal had been to follow my curiosity and zeal to explore a line of study different from my biology and chemistry courses, but what I received from this class was a primer for memorization and a professor who called me a liar to my face.

But back to the final. I aced it and got a B- for the class. While the professor never intimated that my race was a factor in his assessment of me, it was fairly clear that he had never met a student as ethical as me, and my vice dean also felt there may have been racial motivation in his actions. I never interacted with this professor again, but years later, I read a comment he made in an alumni magazine about recognizing new things about teaching at Swarthmore as compared to his other teaching experiences. He stated that he now recognized that one could racially discriminate while teaching a science course. I will never know if he was referring to the horrible treatment I received in his class or some other interaction with a different student.

The great news is that I was able to work at the computer science lab for extra money both at college and in medical school because I took the Intro to Computer Science course. When I needed to use statistical programming in advanced epidemiology training after my dermatology residency, I knew the principles and found this programming quite enjoyable.

Even at a supremely inclusive school like Swarthmore, there are pockets of bias and prejudice that rear their ugly heads. They steal time and thoughts; they leave behind scars that never completely heal. I thought the scary part of going to college was going to be my inadequacy compared to the other students, but the real enemy was prejudice hiding behind the protective walls of education. The only way to survive these experiences is by remembering your ethics, staying on the high road, and doing the work. It's not always easy, but support from friends and family (and administrators at times) can help keep your priorities clear.

If your ethics are called into question or others set out to demean you, dig deep and show your true colors.

Recognizing that microaggressions can appear to derail your progress in school, in work environments, and in interpersonal relationships is key to moving past them and moving forward. If your ethics are called into question or others set out to demean you, dig deep and show your true colors. You may have to work hard to show your worth, and you may need help, but you can overcome these experiences and be successful moving forward. Getting derailed in college or medical school can halt your progress and take you out of the running for competitive awards, recognition for research opportunities, and other accolades, so it's best to address microaggressions as they occur with appropriate responses.

5

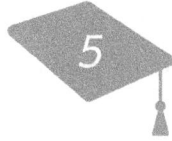

THE INVISIBLES

How Brown and Black People Are Invisible in Medicine

IT MAY SEEM THAT ONCE YOU GET TO MEDICAL SCHOOL, YOU are with your people and all students are on an even playing field, but this is not the case. Medicine, at all levels, can be very competitive, and students who are underrepresented minorities in medicine are often considered to be lesser than. In fact, there are many unwritten rules in clinical medicine that subjugate URiM students compared to majority students. Included in these rules are: faculty not including URiM in discussions of patients during patient rounds, faculty not teaching URiM students on rotations and instead berating them for poor differential diagnoses, faculty giving URiM students poor evaluations at the end of rotations despite never giving advice for improvement, and many more.

Obviously, not all faculty are living by these rules, but enough do that they can be a problem if you are not aware and able to work around them. Not knowing these rules can make it very difficult for students to navigate how to behave appropriately while rotating through their clinical years. Of course, they are adults and should be able to interact with faculty and patients in an ethical manner, but the unwritten rules coupled with a desire to appear prepared can engender competition and poor behavior. In this chapter, I will share some of these rules in order to improve your chance of appearing well-qualified and prepared during interactions with your faculty.

When You Are Not at Home in Medicine

In the first and second year, there are more classes than actual patient rotations. Typically, the early years are spent in the classroom, where students are together in a group with lecturers rather than with faculty one on one on the floors of the hospital or in clinic. There may be interspersed exposures to real patients and preceptors in a clinical setting, but the true clinical rotations where students are part of a team is where their actions can be closely observed.

Any student can find themselves in a new and scary world when they begin doing patient rotations. I remember my first partner for our history-taking experience in medical school. I didn't know this classmate well, but he seemed kind and very bright. He was recognizable because he had a prosthetic leg but was just a regular student in terms of his interactions with others. I didn't know the story behind the prosthesis, but assumed he must've had a lot of medical experiences at some point in his life. I also imagined this would make him very comfortable once we had to go into the hospital to speak to patients. I certainly didn't think that this student would have issue interacting with patients, especially since he was not a URiM student; my experience had been that majority students were confident in all areas of medical training.

At my medical school, we started having interactions much earlier in our training than most medical schools at that time. Nowadays, most medical schools have found that introducing students to patient care early makes better doctors. Back then, my partner and I were to go into a patient's room and simply discuss the reason for their admission. We did not have to perform an examination. It was like a baby step on the way to a full patient–doctor interaction, with just probing questions about their current illness and history of past illness. I thought it was straightforward and very exciting to speak to a real live patient (who had consented to speaking with students).

We entered the room in our crisp bright-white coats, prepared to start asking our questions. We introduced ourselves, then began. "Can you tell us why you are in the hospital, sir?", "What were your symptoms?", "Do take any medications?", and on the questions went. I noticed that I was asking most of the questions, but we hadn't organized who was going to ask what, so I didn't mind. Then I looked up at my classmate, and his face was glistening with sweat. He seemed frozen in place.

It was not clear to me what was happening to my classmate. I thought maybe he was hot or not feeling well. I finished the interview, and we said our goodbyes. Once we left the room, my interview partner was quiet but seemed fine. A similar reaction occurred the next time we had to interview a patient. Every time we reported to our preceptor, I gave the entire history because my partner was still shaken from the experience, a fact that was never commented on. Not too long after that patient experience, he withdrew from medical school and started a job in the university system outside of the medical center.

It eventually dawned on me that my classmate had severe anxiety when faced with patient interactions. He didn't feel at home in medicine. Perhaps, if there had been more support, he would have been able to overcome his anxiety and stay in medical school. Perhaps he was an underrepresented minority because of his body differences, and this may have played a role in his discomfort in medicine. I am at least glad that no one thought less of him when he left. There was concern for his well-being and a shared hope (by all classmates) that he do well in other endeavors.

Unfortunately, during this same time, when a URiM student did not perform up to expectation, they were often called out as not doing a thorough job in front of the rest of the team and graded poorly, rather than leaders overlooking a less-than-stellar performance. URiM students were not guided behind the scenes. They did not receive support from the class. It seemed as if URiM students were expected to do poorly, and it was no major concern if they were to leave. There were URiM students several classes ahead of us who had been asked to take a leave of absence because of a poor performance. They returned to medical school in our class. When they arrived, they were not welcomed back by anyone other than the other URiM students. They were not heralded for having done the work to return, nor were they supported by the administration when they returned.

There are, of course, times when a student is not fit for medical school, but I haven't always observed fairness in properly guiding students. One of the biggest issues with URiM students is just being ignored when it comes to the patient exposure

> One of the biggest issues with URiM students is just being ignored when it comes to the patient exposure portion of the curriculum.

portion of the curriculum. They are very noticeable because of their skin color but also virtually ignored as a learner. That is, they are ignored until they can be pointed to as an example of what not to do and summarily asked to leave. That almost happened to me, as I will discuss later in the book. The point here is that the URiM student often enters and *remains* someone who feels as if they don't belong. The goal with this book is to help *you* belong and show you how to help *others* feel like they belong too.

> The goal with this book is to help *you* belong and show you how to help *others* feel like they belong too.

Support Organizations to Help

What happens when the URiM student is unsupported—but *not* because they have problems with the curriculum, the patient inter-actions, or the various examinations that must be taken? What happens when the URiM student is not seen as fit to be a physician and is basically ignored simply because they do not fit the stereotypical appearance of the field?

The result of being invisible as a medical student is that you're passed over for research opportunities, special fellowships, and mentorships. Too often URiM students are taught at arm's length, with many lessons omitted, causing the student to attempt to self-teach material that should be taught interactively by someone with experience. The student leaves patient rotations feeling obligated to parse through experiences solo to decide on the best way to approach patient care, not knowing what is truly correct. And the student can feel quite alone because they're paying the same tuition as other students but not getting the same education.

There are ways that Black and brown medical students have supported one another, though this should not be a substitute for being taught by an experienced physician. There are historic organizations, like the Student National Medical Association (SNMA), that help support URiM students. The SNMA was founded in 1964 as a spinoff of the parent organization, the National Medical Association (NMA), which was founded in 1895 for Black and African American physicians when they weren't able to join the American Medical Association. The SNMA has a national and regional presence as well as a local presence at most US medical schools. Students who work with the SNMA benefit from leadership opportunities, community projects, tutoring, mentorships, and research. Organizations like this can help the student feel that they belong. This support helps them become successful in the field.

My Medical School Class Makeup

When I arrived at UPenn Medical School, there were nine other Black students in my class. Over the years, several students joined our class from previous classes due to remediation or other reasons, but we remained a small group of approximately twelve students out of a class of one hundred and fifty students. There were students of Hispanic ethnicity, but many of them where white and not brown, and they tended to blend in with the rest of the white students in the class, so they were not treated as invisible.

Black students stand out visibly because of their color but, paradoxically, are often left out of the discussions on rounds and considerations for leadership opportunities. This invisibility can also translate into poor grades in clinical rotations, which often have subjective grading. Something that I experienced commonly until very recently is not being recognized by white physicians outside of the medical center. I have worked closely with physicians on committees and in small groups, but when they encountered me on the street, they just looked right through me, presumably because many do not know Black people outside of work and would not look for someone of color on a random street. You could imagine that these people are ignoring me or simply don't see me, but this is a phenomenon that many Black and brown physicians experience. Most Black physicians accept this as a rite of passage, but this behavior has a name, and it is microaggression (see chapter 4).

What the SNMA did for the Black students in my medical school was allow us to be seen. We could share our experiences and give each other pointers on where to choose rotations to get the fairest and least discriminatory evaluators. We did have an academic advisor who was a woman of color in the dean's office, but she was not a physician and did not hold a position of power. She met with us intermittently and delivered bad news about grades but rarely provided opportunities other than what was handed down from the medical school leadership. The SNMA, on the other hand, was a supportive organization that helped to plan for a successful future in medicine and reached back to support students coming behind us.

How to Excel in Rotations

This lack of mentorship spurred me to become a lifelong mentor for all levels of learners in medicine. My recommendation to students who are entering the clinical years of medical school is to make sure to be observant when the lead physician on a given clinical rotation gives directives but also pay attention to their body language and behaviors. If you are on a rotation in the hospital or clinic setting, and the physician preceptor often gets patient educational materials at the end of patient visits, it would be helpful for the student to notice this and offer to get the materials. If they need assistance with a procedure that is consistently the same, the student should offer to help. This allows the preceptor to see the student as helpful and tuned in to patient care.

It always amazes me when a student rotating with me watches me, on more than a few occasions, determine that a lesion will require a biopsy, but never offers to help set up or notify the nurse for setup despite seeing the process several times. Students are there to learn, and they will learn so much more if they are part of the process of care. If you see an opportunity to help, do so. If you are worried that you will do the wrong thing, you can always ask if there is something you can do or some way you can help.

> If you see an opportunity to help, do so.

Another pointer I give is asking about cases at times that are natural breaks in the action of patient visits, rather than in the patient room or while in the middle of a busy clinic. I have had students ask questions of me while I am trying to explain treatment to a patient, causing the patient to become confused, not to mention the disruption to the visit overall. That is the mark of an unhelpful student, and one who will be remembered with a negative connotation. Remember, timing is everything!

It may seem obvious that students should either pre-round on patients before regular rounds in the hospital or check the clinic schedule prior to an outpatient rotation, but many students of color have not been given this hint, so I make sure to remind them. I also recommend asking for a mid-rotation evaluation from the teaching physician. This is a way to open a dialogue and review case details that the teaching physician may have skipped over due to busy patient care. A mid-rotation evaluation can also help to define specific actions to work on in the second half, including learning issues like self-reliant learning. Finally, I recommend that the student ask questions about the patient cases—when appropriate, of course.

These things should be taught to all students, but some URiM students find that teaching may focus only on the non-URiM students. When the URiM student asks a question or helps with a procedure, it can change how they are viewed by the teaching physician for the better.

Overcoming Barriers in Clinical Medicine

As a member and former president of the Skin of Color Society, a dermatologic society with a mission to improve the mentorship of the next generation, I have a goal to help URiM students overcome barriers. The society has programs in place for observerships, research experiences, presentation opportunities, and more for students and other trainees. For any student who has interest in skin diseases affecting patients with skin of color, and for any URiM interested in dermatology, this is an organization to join and reap all the benefits of membership.

An important barrier to URiM students having confidence on clinical rotations can be due to their cultural experiences. Often, in Black culture, children are taught that they are better seen than heard, and that they must be deferent to those who are in leadership positions. There may be very hierarchical processes in the family where children are discouraged from speaking their minds. Early medical students may have to train themselves to overcome these patterns.

This was part of my problem in the early years of my medical school experience. I hung back and observed but didn't feel my opinion would be welcomed. It wasn't that I was stifled as a child, but it was clear from my parents that their opinions were the last word. I didn't have experience interjecting statements into conversations unless I was asked. I had to unteach myself this habit and gain confidence that what I'm saying is just as important as comments from others at my learning stage. Since there are times when others will discount what URiM students say, I also had to learn to give myself permission to feel okay about saying something, knowing that I might be dismissed or ignored.

Example of Becoming Visible

Our doctor–patient group of approximately eight students was assigned to work with the dean for the case discussion and rounds in the hospital. By that point, I had been surrounded by the super-smart individuals in my class for seven or eight months. They seemed to know all the answers to every question that was asked, even before the question was finished. They innately felt (or at least seemed) confident enough to ask questions in all settings, including the large classroom sessions.

At the beginning of rounds, the dean began describing a case of a little boy brought to the emergency room by his mother. He had begun to have muscle rigidity and listlessness, lasting for several days. He had been well prior to these symptoms, and no one else in the family was ill. The dean asked what questions we would ask of the patient's mother. The students on my team were surprisingly quiet. They seemed to be out of their element when the question wasn't textbook-related and an actual patient was involved.

For me, this kind of medical dilemma was why I wanted to be a doctor. I loved the medical show called *Dr. Marcus Welby, MD*. I loved his life as a physician where he seemed to be able to solve any medical mystery, from sudden onset seizures to a new skin rash. The idea of solving this medical mystery was right up my alley. To my own surprise, I spoke up. I asked if the patient had eaten something different from the rest of the family or had stayed at another location where his exposures were different than usual. The answers to my questions were "no" and "no," but I saw a gleam in the dean's eye when I asked my questions, as if I was onto something. Another student chimed in with a question, but the other students remained silent. The dean told us the diagnosis: botulism, a bacterial infection from a cut he sustained from a metal can in his yard. The dean asked me and the other student who spoke up to write a short report on the mechanism of muscle rigidity in botulinum toxicity.

While most people would not look at extra work as a gift, it was a message to me that I was seen. That is a lesson I would have to learn several times in medicine. When others in leadership positions ask you to write a report, case, or research manuscript, that means they think highly enough of you to want to mentor you in your medical career.

Reach a balance in clinical rotations, somewhere between being outspoken and confident versus being over-confident and obnoxious.

For most of my mentees, invisibility is not desirable. You must reach a balance in clinical rotations, somewhere between being outspoken and confident versus being over-confident and obnoxious. It is better to be subtle rather than forceful.

6

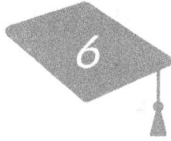

WHAT THE WHITE MEN SAY

Who Defines Your Worth in Medicine

IN MY EARLIEST YEARS, MY WORLD WAS LIMITED TO BROWN people. Everyone in my neighborhood and in my family were African American. As I got older and matriculated into a private school in the fourth grade, I had to learn to exist in a space where the majority was white. As I think now about how I learned to exist in this majority white environment, I recognize that white men have typically defined every space.

There have been a lot of white men in my social and work life. The first were work colleagues of my father, then a white principal of my elementary school, and many in my private school until twelfth grade, at college, in medical school, in my dermatology residency, in my additional epidemiology training, and in my academic career at my medical center. Perhaps it is no surprise that white men are in these spaces, since they have, historically, been leaders in them.

The surprise to me is that I can make a statement that is well founded and important that will not be taken seriously until a white man in the room says it. There is a well-known method of women empowering the words of other women by repeating a statement made by a woman and attributing the statement to the original speaker, thereby giving credence to the comment. Men, of course, do not typically need this trick to be heard.

There are many other strategic ways women must learn to be heard in the classroom, the board room, the faculty meeting, etc. I have used some of these techniques successfully; others less so. The one thing that continues to amaze me is that when white men I don't know well address me, I still have to consider their comments on several levels. Is this kind statement a back-handed way to put me down? Is this unkind comment being said because I am a woman, because I am Black, because I am short? As a full professor and former chair of a department, it is astonishing that I need to consider all these questions before I can formulate a coherent and appropriate response.

> There are many strategic ways women must learn to be heard in the classroom, the board room, the faculty meeting, etc.

When Others Define Your Race

One of the first white men who told me something that made me pause was in medical school. I was in York, Pennsylvania, for a medical school rotation in obstetrics and gynecology. York is a bucolic historic town approximately one and a half hours outside of Philadelphia, and we rotated at the teaching hospital there. We stayed in a dorm-like situation and had communal meals in the cafeteria (with the most delicious food that I had ever eaten at a cafeteria). It was away from distractions, so there was time for studying and long conversations with our fellow students. The hospital was located across from the York campus with beautiful tree-lined trails that invited me to run several miles a week, even though I am not a runner. This atmosphere was in direct contrast to the many thirteen- and fourteen-year-old pregnant girls we were taking care of in the maternity ward, many of whom were white.

This conversation in question was with a fellow medical student who was on a different rotation at the hospital. He and I were discussing something that led him to make a comment about how I was different from other Black people. I don't remember what was said to make him share this, but it wasn't the first time I'd heard it. I'd heard it on television and in classrooms before this. He told me that the Black people who made it to medical school were different from other Black people who didn't do well in school and who were on drugs or having babies in high school.

I let him know that there is little difference between me and others in my very own neighborhood who may have been less successful. I explained that the difference was not the person, but the opportunities given to them. It had been my parents, and what they made available to me and my sister as we grew up, that changed our perspective. They showed us how exciting it was for us to learn and do well in school. They made sure that we understood that education equaled success. My classmate did not see how it could be as simple as this. He told me that Black people needed to have a leader, someone like Martin Luther King, Jr., to lead them out of crime and toward education.

> The difference is not the person, but the opportunities given to them.

I asked him who the leader of the white people was, and he said the US president. I asked him why the president was not the leader of all people, no matter what the color, and he did not have an answer to that question. I was not advanced enough in my thinking to interject the topic of bias and generational structural racism into our conversation as the real challenge for many people of color. But this discourse prepared me for the narrow thinking that I would encounter time and time again in my travels through medical training and beyond.

Differential Treatment as a Medical Student of Color

When I was a third-year medical student on hospital rotations, there was a medicine resident on my internal medicine service who never called me to work up a patient unless I called him multiple times throughout the evening. The rule was that third-year medical students were not to stay overnight on call and were to be called by 8:00 p.m. in order to meet and examine a patient before heading out by 11:00 p.m. This tall, cocky white man, who had been described by our attending physician (the senior physician leading the team) as a "boy wonder," was anything but that for me. Since he never called me (there were no cell phones at this time and students did not have pagers), I would page him at intervals. He invariably told me at my 10:00 p.m. or 11:00 p.m. call that there was patient for me, though the patient was admitted many hours earlier. I had to complete my workup later than required and then head home to write my report until the wee hours of the night, making me just a bit less sharp than I would have liked.

My roommate, who was white, was called by her resident as early as possible with her patient of the night so she could have time to look up any important details about the case before morning report. At the resident's instruction, she would call him and go over the case to make sure she covered all the salient features of the exam and illness. My resident, on the other hand, would tell me *not* to call him with questions and that I would be fine on my own. This was bias at its clearest.

The differential teaching could have made me an inferior physician if I hadn't been such a conscientious student and if I didn't have the network of Black students who supported each other in these situations. I checked with other students after my rotation with this resident to see if he treated all medical students this way, and indeed, he did not treat white students this way during their rotations.

This same resident once told me that an extremely high thyroid hormone level I found on one of the patients I was following was "not a big deal." When I looked up the value, it seemed quite high to me. Luckily, a senior resident from another team was standing nearby and heard our discussion. He interjected that the value was the highest he had ever seen. My resident took the chart from me as I was documenting the finding and wrote the note up himself as if he had found the lab value. I always wondered what this guy thought he was winning by trying to deprive me of the correct medical practices. Did he just think it would help me fail later? Was he so biased that he did not want the patients I treated to get better? Experiences like this ultimately helped me decide to go into academic medicine. I wanted to make sure that *all* students received excellent teaching, no matter their racial background. I also wanted majority

I want to make sure that *all* students receive excellent teaching, no matter their racial background.

students (non-minority students) to understand that doctors of color could be their teachers.

Recognizing an Unbiased and Unprejudiced Training Program

By the time I got to my dermatology residency after medical school and my one-year Internal Medicine internship, I was ready for anything. I had been the recipient and the observer of so many micro-aggressions and macroaggressions (though they weren't called that then) that I was ready for them. My attitude was "Bring it on!" To my surprise, I sensed a new dynamic almost immediately after starting my residency at the University of Michigan (U of M).

At the time, back in 1990, the U of M dermatology program was one of the top, if not *the* top, dermatology programs, and I assumed it would be like my experience in medical school at the University of Pennsylvania, with few faculty of color and consistent microaggressions. It was considered a large dermatology residency program with eighteen to twenty residents when most residencies had six to nine residents, and the dynamic was more of a resident versus faculty power struggle. At that time, the U of M program was very clear on valuing residents of color, so there were always two or three Black residents in the program. As a matter of fact, John Kenny, the first Black dermatology chair of a department, had trained at Michigan, and U of M was quite proud of this fact.

When I arrived, my class was quite diverse: me, a Puerto Rican woman, an Asian woman, a white woman, and two white men. The power struggle, as the year went on, was clearly the faculty sending messages from on high and the residents trying to take back control of their schedules, their rotation locations, and even the number of medical meetings we were approved to attend. There was grumbling about the chair and the residency program director—so many complaints about so many things, I couldn't keep track. But I was happy because there was no racial discrimination from the leadership. When the residents were treated poorly, we were all treated poorly in the same way, so I couldn't figure out what the other residents were complaining about. This was heaven for me. I was not getting differential medical training because of the color of my skin. That was a bonus in my book, though it should have been simply an expectation.

I did feel the pressure to be excellent. One of the senior Black residents shared that we, as Black residents, needed to perform at the highest level possible. This was nothing new to me as I had learned that as one of few Blacks in any situation, the microscope is always on our behavior.

The U of M department was all white men, and the things that they said and did were supportive of my career and were, I believe, a big part of the reason I achieved success in my academic career. The chair, Dr. John Voorhees, and the program director, Dr. Chuck Ellis, not to mention several other key faculty members, were big supporters of my career. After residency, they invited me back for lectureships in the department as well as to medical meetings. I will never forget that support, and it spurs me to pay it forward with my students and residents.

As a faculty member at Wake Forest, I had one of the most supportive mentors of my career in my corner. My founding and former chair, Dr. Joe Jorizzo, is a white man and one of the most openminded and supportive mentors in my life. He did not realize that I was Black until I arrived for my interview, and he was even more excited once he found out. That was certainly a topsy-turvy world for me. As time went on, he nurtured my academic interests, helped direct my focus, and steered me clear of the many pitfalls in academic medicine. I achieved many of my career goals with his support and the support of others in the field of dermatology—which is, for the most part, a welcoming specialty.

Microaggressions May Never Stop and How to Handle Them

When I ventured outside of my department in my own institution, I didn't find quite as much support. Most of the time, as a chair of the department, other chairs were helpful and supportive. But there were a few who seemed to lack the supportive gene. One chair in particular was always spouting off about his latest conquest for his department or his collection of toys (Tesla, Apple Watch, new interactive conference room update, etc.). In March 2020, the southeastern part of the United States was just heading into the COVID-19 pandemic, and we began to have our weekly chair meetings virtually. The meetings were discussions where any chairs could come and discuss interesting leadership information or just commiserate about necessary tasks. We started talking about COVID.

I had been reading the data out of China and talking to my fellow dermatology chairs in New York, Boston, and Detroit, where they were far ahead of the curve of active cases. They described how they left work one day with the edict that masks were not allowed and returned the next to be told that masks were mandated. This was before widespread mask mandates. In the weekly meeting, I stated that we would all soon be wearing masks. And the very vocal, conquest-bragging chair told me, as if speaking to a five-year-old, "Amy, we will *not* be wearing masks because there are not enough PPE (personal protective equipment) for everyone," and that this was not going to happen for a variety of other reasons. I held my ground, but not a single person on the call (all white men) came to my defense. We all know how that story ended: with wide-spread international mask mandates.

Even though I was exactly at his level and was well respected in my field, this man still felt comfortable telling me off. This behavior was on brand for his personality, but the others not pulling for me was a bit of a gut punch. It served to remind me that I may exist in this world of academic medicine, but I am not always viewed as a card-carrying member by others. There may have been some bystander surprise, and perhaps that stopped the others from saying anything. However, this experience serves as a good example of something that happens to women and members of minority groups frequently.

The lesson here is to stand your ground when others question your thinking. If you are sure that you have made a reasonable comment, stay calm, make your point again, and then leave it. There is no need to drive home to the dissenting person that you are right because often, as in this case, time will do all the work for you.

Stand your ground when others question your thinking.

7

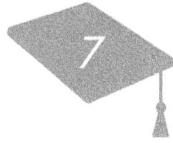

Perform Like Beyoncé

How You Can Perform at Your Highest Level

Just imagine you are in a huge concert venue and the music is starting. You have just seen an amazing warm-up act; you're ready to see the main act. You paid top dollar to see a mind-blowing performer. The lights finally dim. The music from their most popular song starts, and the performer appears on stage. They hang their head and hum along with the music, but they never start singing or dancing and the music just plays. This would be a horrible outcome to what you hoped would be an amazing experience. And this is how patients feel when you do not bring your full energy to their visit.

After all, would you want to just chalk up a bad performance of your favorite artist to "having a bad day"? Would you be okay with paying your money and just getting an average-to-poor performance? Would you care if the performer had a bad night's sleep or some concerning news the day before their concert? Imagine if the performer were Beyoncé and she came out and just walked through her dance steps and hummed her songs instead of singing. I don't think *anyone* would accept this lack of performance. Being a professional means that if you are at work or school and you are well, you will deliver what is needed during your rotations. Of course, everyone gets tired or has family issues, but you must put your all into your work and leave everything on the floor when you are in clinical rotation!

When you are on a rotation and you show up late or unprepared or have no idea what you are doing because you didn't complete the prereading, you show everyone on the rotation that you're not up to a full performance—*even* if you were good last week and the week before. The same is true for patient care. The patient in the room is paying hard-earned money to receive a service. They don't care if you had car trouble yesterday or if your cat has digestive issues and you lost a night of sleep. They just want you to be present to listen to their story and perform an appropriate and thorough exam, followed by designing a full treatment recommendation. This is how physicians "leave it all on the floor." If you can't do this most days, patients and coworkers alike will be able to tell.

What Not to Do on Rotation

Some years ago, I had a physician assistant student assigned to me for a rotation. He was a bit older than the typical PA student because he had worked for several years before starting PA school. I figured his past work experience would make him a great student, but this wasn't the case. The first day of clinic, the student shadowed me. During my interactions with patients, the student immediately sat down in any available chair in the patient room. If there was no chair available, he leaned on whatever he could find. At the end of a very busy clinic, he asked me how I could stand for so long and have stamina to move from room to room so quickly. He came to clinic unprepared for the work and was tired and dragging after three hours.

Luckily, this student was not interested in dermatology, so I didn't have to have the difficult discussion about how he was not a good fit for the specialty. But I did have to evaluate his performance on the rotation. As you might imagine, he received a poor evaluation from me; he did not perform as well as he could have, and he definitely did not "leave it all on the floor" during the clinic.

When you are on rotation, you need to bring it! Bring your energy, bring your curiosity, bring your innovation, bring your humor, bring your team spirit, and most of all, bring your interest in the topic at hand.

> Bring your energy, bring your curiosity, bring your innovation, bring your humor, bring your team spirit, and most of all, bring your interest in the topic at hand.

How to Perform Well on Rotation

The flip side of not being prepared on rotation is being ready to face whatever may come. The best students are those who preview the patient list before they arrive on site. They are appropriately dressed and don't come with too many snacks or large bags that take up room in the tight confines of a clinic workroom. They keep their water or coffee in a safe place away from the fray of clinic.

When clinic begins, the excellent students ask for direction on what patients they can see and how you'd like the case presented. They only ask once and get it right the rest of the time they work with that particular physician. They spend a short time in the patient room obtaining the history in order to keep the clinic on time, and they have a cohesive report on what is happening with the patient and a brief exam along with a consideration of diagnosis and treatment. In dermatology, for instance, the important thing for students is to be able to describe lesions using primary lesion descriptors (i.e., papules, macules, pustules, nodules, vesicles), rather than saying "lesions" or "bumps." This is even more important than knowing the diagnosis. It's much more impressive if a student can master this terminology because it is how we formulate diagnoses and will give me more to go on than aimless descriptions of "spots."

An example of this mastery was when a dermatology resident from another country came to work with me for a few months. She was obviously more experienced than a student, and she was so organized in her presentations and her thinking that she actually helped me complete clinic early. I have had a few students like this as well, so that is the aspirational experience for a student.

One faux pas that students can make is to feel that they must lie about the history of exam if they are asked about a skin finding or a historical aspect of the case. If a faculty member asks you, the student, a question about something that you didn't look at or ask about, please answer truthfully. When you are not truthful and the faculty member recognizes this, you lose credibility about *everything*. I wouldn't want a dishonest doctor, and I don't want to train people who are dishonest.

One recent student gave a reasonable presentation about a patient who was coming for increased pigmentation on the face. She had been seen in the past for a severe form of hair loss, and this was available to him on the old note. Once he completed the presentation, I asked him if he looked at her scalp. He said yes. I asked what he saw, and he answered that he did not see anything of consequence. But the patient had complete hair loss. I immediately knew this student was dishonest, and I simply put him in the category of someone that I didn't want to train long term. Don't be this person. Tell the truth! If you didn't look at the area or ask the historical question, just say that. No one is perfect, and that is understood, but lying is a repugnant and a bad practice in medicine.

No one is perfect, and that is understood, but lying is a repugnant and a bad practice in medicine.

Prepared students arrive early to clinic. They are kind to the patients and succinct in their explanations of the patient history. They are praised by patients for their thoroughness. They leave clear and brief notes on the intake sheet for me to use while I am writing my notes. They are not trying to be my best friend by being too familiar; they always remain professional. This is how a student can "leave it all on the floor" during the rotation.

Even at the level of residency, you will need to continue to bring your enthusiasm. There was a resident I will call Bruce who came to work one Monday morning to work with me in my clinic. First, he said he was exhausted, then he put his head down on the desk near his computer. When the first patient was ready, he got up slowly, as if he could barely stand. I asked him why he was so tired and if he was ill. Bruce told me that he had a rough weekend. He said that he had broken up with his girlfriend a few days before the weekend and she had taken all her furniture out of his apartment. I can certainly understand being sad about a break-up and not being 100%, but there is a limit to how much of this you bring to work. You can break down at lunch or after work with your friends, but again, patients don't care if you had a breakup or if your girlfriend took all her furniture. And if you are not well and cannot perform up to par, it is time to take a short time off to get your head clear so you can return full strength.

This same is true for deaths in the family and pet deaths. You are not a robot, and everyone has loss. No one expects you to be happy and peppy when you have faced sad issues in your family. The key is that you need to be professional in how you handle these hard times when they arise. You need to utilize your support system and get those feelings out, but then you must pull it together for work. If you can't do this, medicine will be a very difficult career choice for you. Part of being a professional is recognizing when you need help—and taking time to get it.

Part of being a professional is recognizing when you need help—and taking time to get it.

Know Your Limits in Order to Perform at Your Highest Level

I had a very sweet young medical student who was scheduled to work with me for several weeks. She attended a different medical school than where I work, and she had a two-week block set up with me as well as another two-week rotation with a dermatologist at yet another medical center. A week before she was to arrive, she contacted me to say that her mother had passed away. When she told me this, I immediately suggested that we cancel so she could take time to grieve and spend the time with family. She insisted that she should come anyway. She stated that mother's friends were encouraging her to continue her scheduled rotations and to attend to her responsibilities as a student. I knew it was a bad idea, but she was determined, so I let her come. I did not know her well, and I thought I would give her an opportunity to shine, even in the worst of circumstances.

The student came and was sad and grieving, as I expected. She was unable to work through a full clinic without breaking down into tears. I recommended that she leave early each day and go back to her hotel. I finally encouraged her to leave the rotation early, so she could grieve with family without having to worry about trying to perform.

This was a case of a student trying her best to work—but also someone who couldn't assess her own grief and limitations. I wouldn't have thought ill of this student if she had cancelled her rotation, and I didn't think ill of her when she left the rotation early, but I did feel a bit frustrated that she didn't listen to me in the first place. I lost my mother as well, so I know what that feels like. For me, work was a balm that helped me take my mind off being sad, but I had the benefit of being much older than this student, and I was already a practicing physician at the time of my mother's death. Students who are still learning and do not have the practice experience that I had may not manage loss as easily at work. It's important to give yourself grace and take time to grieve in a way that feels right for you. Everyone handles grief in their own way, but you need to be self-aware enough to know when you can perform like Beyoncé and when you need to take a break.

It is important to find support if you realize you can't pull yourself together after a great loss. If your usual friends and family are not enough, you need to find out where you can get additional help. Medical school is not easy, and when your health (mental or otherwise) is at risk, it may be the time for school to be put on the back burner. Sometimes, pulling yourself up by your bootstraps isn't going to work. That's when you gather all your resources together, even if that means taking time off. Asking for help is not a bad thing, nor is taking time to get back to your most productive self. In such times, it is important to have mentors and supports in place to help you get back on a successful path.

I had a resident who, unfortunately, had to face a divorce early in her time in the residency. The breakup was long and drawn out, and this resident had a hard time compartmentalizing her feelings about the loss. She was often late to teaching sessions and distracted in clinics. As chair of the department at the time, I insisted she see Employee Assistance for help. She didn't love the idea at first, but she managed to go for help and things started to improve. Whether it was timing or the outside assistance she received, she turned over a new leaf and got her head back in the game at work. She finished her residency strong and has been very successful as a dermatologist with a lovely new spouse and young children.

Seeing the light at the end of the tunnel is not easy when you are facing a devastating loss—but in normal times, there is no excuse. When you cannot perform at a high level, ask yourself what you need to do for self-care and take time to heal. Get outside help if needed and don't assume you can do everything on your own. Once you are fully healed, get ready to bring it like Beyoncé. Your patients and healthcare colleagues alike will appreciate your attentiveness to detail and care.

Get outside help if needed and don't assume you can do everything on your own.

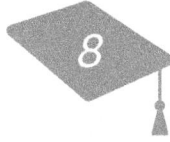

How Communicating
Clearly Can Help You

WHEN YOU'RE A MEDICAL STUDENT OR AN EARLY LEARNER IN medicine, your voice is not as easily heard as those leading healthcare teams. There's a hierarchy in medicine that has been present since the beginning of organized medicine. Therefore, making a good impression on patient rounds, in patient presentations, during research, and in mentor meetings is difficult. You have a short time to shine, so communicating clearly and well is paramount.

As a student, your written and oral communication is important. Once you become a physician, one of the expected skills is to be able to deliver a clear and enjoyable discussion about your area of expertise. You may not have to do this frequently if you are solely in private practice and not interested in academic medicine, but many physicians of all types become involved in boards of companies or consultancies where communication is important.

The biggest need for clear communication is, of course, with patients. You may be the smartest person in your class, but if you can't speak in a way that patients understand, you won't be successful in clinical medicine.

Good Communication May Be Natural or Learned

Little time is allotted in medical school to teach good communication skills. For some, speaking eloquently comes naturally. They're born with the gene for being an effective speaker, covering topics with ease. I believe those people self-select for academic medicine, so it is not a surprise that you'll meet lots of them. There are many of us who *don't* come by this skill naturally. I wasn't gifted with the speaking gene. I was someone who had to work at being proficient at talks.

One of the first truths for someone who is an awkward speaker *and* who wants to become a dynamic speaker, whether as a student on rounds or a presenter at a medical meeting, is that motivation and some enjoyment of at least part of the process are necessary. Those who have significant panic and anxiety with oral presentations should work on this first. Even motivation will not make this better. Specific relaxation techniques or anxiolytic medications might be required, but most people are teachable.

There are many options for those who are working on being better communicators. Online and in-person programs and books can help with communication. Students can have friends and mentors help them practice presentations, giving feedback on their delivery, tone, and body language. It can be helpful to start with a taping of how you look while presenting and evaluating what works and what doesn't.

The point is that everyone can benefit from refining their oral delivery, so adding this to the list of to-dos is a good idea.

Putting Yourself Out There as a Speaker or Communicator

My first lecture experience was during my residency. My program director asked me to stand in for one of the faculty lecturers who was out of town. Our program required each resident to give a talk using slides, and I had recently completed mine. I had delivered the initial talk to my fellow residents and a few attending faculty members, so I was comfortable. This time, the talk was going to be to the entire second-year medical school class of over one hundred students. Even though I felt comfortable that I knew more dermatology than these students, I still felt anxiety about several things: standing at the podium alone, teaching well enough for the students to understand my lectures, and measuring up to previous lecturers.

I practiced and practiced, then delivered the lecture to the students, and it seemed to go fine. I couldn't tell if the students got anything out of it, but I felt I had really accomplished something and was energized by the experience. Right after the talk, I exited the lecture hall to find ten medical students—most of whom were students of color—excited and asking questions about the specialty of dermatology. They hadn't seen many people of color in their curriculum and perhaps never considered that Black people could be dermatologists. I had accomplished more than I thought. I had delivered medical knowledge on a big stage, but I also activated students to consider a career choice they might never have considered.

The knowledge that I could encourage others to think beyond the bounds of their imagination was heady stuff. It was a bit addictive, but in a good way. It helped me recognize that having some aspect of teaching in my future career would energize me. It was also a stepping stone to choosing an academic career and a good example of saying "yes" to something I may not have wanted to do at first. It turns out, one of those medical students in my lecture charted a course to dermatology and is a successful dermatologist today.

Something that is often lost on those who are not members of a minority group, especially for URiM individuals, is that we are rarely regarded as having enough authority for others to learn from us. Most white physicians don't have to consider if they will be taken seriously as an expert in medicine. It is quite acceptable, and perhaps expected, for people of color to be expert in music, dance, or sports, but the medical world is not as accepting.

I tried to explain this to a vice dean in our medical school some years ago. A new rule was put into place to allow only one lecturer from each department for the medical student curriculum. We had a wonderful faculty member who was white running the course for our department, but many of the faculty in the department historically lectured in the course. It was understandable on one level that the lectures were being restricted to the course director because this prevented rogue lecturers who only wanted to talk about their rare research issues rather than teach the students what they needed for patient care. The unplanned consequence was that the students would no longer see a Black, female, full professor in front of them as a person of authority.

When I explained this the vice dean, who was a very self-confident and almost arrogant white woman, she suggested that instead of lecturing in the course, I speak to the students about my journey in medicine. She couldn't see that this offer was nothing like being the authority on the subject matter that was going to be tested. I declined her offer. The students who wanted to learn about my journey seemed to find me on their own. This is the unwritten loss that occurs without a concerted effort to balance the curriculum with diverse teachers.

The Art of Public Speaking

Nowadays, students are often in a position to give lectures, typically at the end of rotations or by presenting their research at meetings. Needing to comport yourself well during a presentation comes earlier in the process of medical training than in the past. For many students who take a research year during medical school, it is important to become comfortable delivering short, engaging lectures about your research.

It is important to become comfortable delivering short, engaging lectures about your research.

In terms of the art of public speaking in medicine, those with simple generalized lack of confidence or ability *can* learn. My personal issue regarding public speaking is that I am an introvert who has tapped into other areas of my brain to act more like an extrovert when it comes to seeing patients, but the extrovert behavior did *not* include an approach to public speaking. Once I realized that I could expand the extroverted part of my personality, it was easier to practice being a more vibrant speaker.

I realized early on in my faculty career that my lectures were acceptable, but not great. I took it upon myself to watch the masters and learn. I attended enough medical meetings that I could see rhythms in brilliant talks, each specialty having a slightly different cadence. The best speakers transcend the specialty rhythm and give an outstanding talk to *any* audience. That was my goal. I did a few key things to push myself down the road to outstanding.

> The best speakers transcend the specialty rhythm and give an outstanding talk to *any* audience.

After I became a student of the master speakers, I decided I needed to truly study the art of speaking with a textbook. I reviewed several books but found one to be most suited to the way I learn. It was a simple book called *Talk Like Ted*, by Carmine Gallo.[12] This book taught me to think about my audience in an innovative way. It helped me humanize my message while still delivering practical information. I read this book many years ago, but the salient points are ingrained in each lecture I deliver.

I determine my main points prior to building the lecture. I pick the number of slides that fit the time allotted. (It's always disappointing when the speaker says that they'll rush through slides because time has run out. It still happens to me occasionally, but never in major talks.) I always add something that is surprising and thought provoking so the talk is memorable. I practice my new talks for time and emphasis, and I try to finish making my talks before the deadline to have a few days away before I finalize my slides. I have also worked on my delivery to make it fit the venue.

I still make many other tweaks because I'm always on a quest to improve, and I'm always learning.

For students, you'll need to be able to communicate well both verbally and in writing. If you work with others for research, you'll need to write a reasonable outline and paper. Good communication can help you be noticed during residency interviews and in clinic when your presentations are succinct and helpful for the faculty. You may need help with this, perhaps from a mentor or other student colleagues. For oral presentations, you may think you have a handle on the material, but you need to complete your presentation well in advance of the due date to allow time for you to present for your mentor and allow for corrections and additions. Remember that you are representing your mentor when you are speaking publicly, and you want to make them proud as well as allow others to appreciate their excellent mentorship of you.

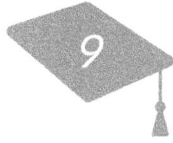

LEADERSHIP IN MEDICAL SCHOOL

LEADERSHIP CAN TAKE MANY FORMS, AND MEDICAL SCHOOL is a great place to get a taste of just how important it can be as you move through your career as a physician. Most medical students have shown leadership qualities as an undergraduate, which likely contributed to why they were admitted to medical school in the first place. But you must not think of medical school as the end goal. In so many ways, it's just the beginning. And how you chart your course through medical school will determine how successful you are during your residency—and ultimately your practice of medicine.

I see medical students all the time who consider that "P" (as in PASS) equals MD. In other words, the thinking is that all you need to do is the minimum to pass, and that's enough. After all, it's medical school—that's the trophy at the end of the game, right? Wrong! While most medical schools are now pass/fail, you need to consider more than just achieving passing grades. Being a great doctor takes more than measurable lessons. It takes recognizing the needs of the community you serve. It takes reaching back and helping those who are coming behind you. And

Put yourself in the shoes of the patient and think of what kind of doctor you would want in a physician.

it takes broadening your own perspective on medicine, whether that is with research, volunteerism, advocacy, or other pursuits. Put yourself in the shoes of the patient and think of what kind of doctor you would want in a physician.

How Not to Approach Medical School

I spoke with one third-year student who contacted me about applying to dermatology residency. She was referred to me by a faculty member in another department. As I questioned her about her extracurricular activities, she stated that she made a conscious decision to focus on being a student while in medical school. She did absolutely nothing other than study and complete the required work for school. Her choice was great for her, but she didn't seem to understand that it wouldn't fly for competitive residencies. She stated that she felt that her record in classes and the required activities should be enough. I am not sure why this student felt that her own personal decisions would be applicable to advanced training programs with which she had no experience. She told me that she would be most interested in attending residency at our medical center. When I mentioned that there were many students who had been involved with the department since their first year and that these students were a known quantity and she was not, she simply ignored me. I tried to explain that there is no way to support a student who has no history with the department in terms of letters of recommendation. She seemed to feel that she was an excellent candidate even without this exposure.

This student was not only sorely mistaken, but she was so poorly informed about the process of applying into dermatology that she made a memorably bad first impression with someone who has been in leadership in a dermatology department for thirty years. This is *clearly* not a good way to begin a career in the specialty that you hope to pursue. It's also the antithesis of leadership. It's simply checking the boxes that are set in front of you and expecting something good to come of it. Sure, she's fine regarding her *medical school* career, and this may be fine for a less competitive residency than dermatology. However, no residency wants a resident who cannot be bothered to go the extra mile for their chosen specialty, and certainly no one wants a doctor who just completes the status quo at work.

Defining Leadership for Medical Students

What is important is recognizing that taking the lead in an area outside of the classroom allows you to grow as a person. Some students have traveled a great distance to get to medical school, so they are natural leaders. For instance, some students are the first in their family to go to college. Some are immigrants to the United States who basically had to fend for themselves for many years before even applying for college.

Often, students with backgrounds like this will recognize where there is a need that they can fulfill. It might be in volunteering in the student-run free clinic associated with their medical school and ultimately

> Taking the lead in an area outside of the classroom allows you to grow as a person.

becoming the head of the free clinic student leadership. They might find that they're best suited to volunteer in the community with the Boys or Girls Club of America or at their local church.

Leadership in volunteerism looks great on a CV, but more importantly, it gives back to the community and allows you to grow and mature. The knowledge of how to care for those who are not fortunate enough to have healthcare shows an understanding of the world that is attractive to residency programs, most of which staff some variant of free clinics as well.

Other options that I have observed in students who lead include research leadership, student government leadership, tutoring, business development, and even leadership in the arts. Some students are dancers and keep this going throughout medical school, either founding or joining dance troupes, or they write for various outlets, or they sing in a capella groups, or they may even teach yoga or other exercise classes. Truly, the sky is the limit for ways to excel. Any of these options shows that you're not stagnant and that you're continuing to improve and grow as a person while helping others. Less important is which you pick; it only matters that you pick *something* and be part of this activity longitudinally, and it helps if you pick something that you enjoy and want to pursue. You should do what you're passionate about because it shows if you're not.

An Example of Student Leadership

One dermatology applicant who stands out in my mind as a leader is a young physician who had chosen to pursue a specialty other than dermatology. He had completed residency and was already a faculty member in this specialty at another institution. This young man approached me after I had given a talk at a medical meeting. He asked if we could talk about getting into dermatology. I gave him my card and recommended that he email me, which he did, and we set up a time to talk.

He was a softspoken person but was quite perceptive and aware of the difficulties he would face in attempting to change from one specialty to another, especially after already completing a full residency. He shared that he had found his current specialty interesting but had always thought about dermatology. He had found crossover cases with dermatology in his current specialty and was already having some success working with one dermatologist in his medical center with these cases. That was leadership quality number one—he had already reached out to the department to start his journey. He also shared that he had a leadership role in his department during COVID, so that was leadership quality number two.

Over the course of approximately six months, this young physician and I set out goals he needed to work toward. They included scheduling meetings with the chair of the department and the program director, finding more ways to work with the person with whom he was already collaborating, spending more time in the department for conferences, and talking with the current dermatology residents about the program. The young man strategically completed all the tasks we laid out and had a successful match for dermatology one year later. It was clear that taking the lead on his career trajectory was attractive to programs, as he was offered several residency interviews based on his accomplishments.

Leadership in this case did not mean that he had to be the head of a dermatologic organization, just that he was showing his abilities and offering his talents to improve knowledge in the specialty.

Self-Awareness as a Tool for Leadership

Another young physician who impressed me with her leadership abilities is a young woman I met when she was a fourth-year medical student from another medical school. She contacted me about coming to work with me, and we settled on her applying for a mentorship grant through a dermatology organization. She immediately completed the application and was ultimately awarded the position.

When this young woman arrived, we talked about her journey to medical school. Her story was an amazing tale of survival. Her American father had met her mother in Africa and brought her back to live with him in the United States, even though he was already married. They had two children together but were never able to provide well for the family. It turned out that he was also running several shady business deals that ended poorly, leaving him in jail and her mother deported. My young mentee went to live with her paternal grandmother, who was able to provide the necessities and the support she and her sibling needed to go to school. My mentee was observant and noted that there were other ways to live that were more comfortable than how she was raised. She vowed to get a college and medical school education to help achieve her goals. She became the leader of her own life.

Once in medical school on scholarship, she found dermatology, but after attending a dermatologic conference where other students were presenting their work, she quickly realized that she was not at a level that would be competitive for matching in the specialty. That was when she reached out to me and several other leaders of color in the specialty. I was committed to helping her achieve her goals to increase her knowledge of the specialty and work on a research project, and she was an excellent learner. She completed a project with me in record time, as well as another four visiting dermatology rotations at other medical schools when it became clear that her own institution wouldn't support her quest. To save money, this young woman literally drove across the country twice to get to all the rotations and back to her own school to complete her requirements. She showed grit and leadership, and those qualities helped her match into a dermatology residency position, making all her mentors proud.

The moral of these stories is that you can utilize the recommendations and counsel of a trusted leader in your specialty of choice to help elevate you to the next level. Becoming a leader early in your career will expand your reach for immediate goals (residency interviews), but more importantly, it will expand your reach to be a recognized and respected part of the medical community.

> Utilize the recommendations and counsel of a trusted leader in your specialty of choice to help elevate you to the next level.

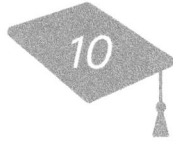

TO RESEARCH OR
NOT TO RESEARCH

IT'S NO SECRET THAT MEDICAL STUDENTS ARE WORRIED about the need to complete research projects when they are interested in matching into a competitive residency like dermatology. The question isn't just whether you need to complete research but also how much research you should do and what level of authorship you should have.

I have had many medical students contact me *frantic* to get a research project in dermatology. Often, their medical school doesn't have a dermatology department or there are no adequate research opportunities. They've heard that research counts for a lot, so they become hyperfocused on getting one or more research projects completed. When I speak to these students, they often have no plan for how to fit research into their curriculum, and many have not considered their overall accomplishments and whether research is the right place to start for building a curriculum vitae.

Don't Panic, Assess

The first thing to do when considering dermatology research is to stop panicking. Not every person who has matched in dermatology has performed true research, but it has certainly come to be expected for applicants to have done at least a bit of research. However, if you decide not to write anything (a case or case series or online publication), this means you need to have an amazing application in every other way. Even one publication of a case can show that you tried your best, if a full-fledged research project is not possible. If you attend a medical school that has research programs, it will seem that you've missed an opportunity if you don't try a bit of research.

For medical students in general, research definitely elevates your application, but for dermatology-bound students, it's very important to approach research as something *achievable*. You have to understand where you are starting and what you can master while in school. If you've never performed research before, you will need to find a mentor who is willing to help you. If you *have* been involved in lots of research in the past, you may be able to really fly—but guess what! You will also need a mentor to help you. The common denominator is a good mentor.

In the last few years, eager medical students have reached out to me in the early part of their first year to talk about research. They know that dermatology is competitive and want to get an early start. I usually recommend that students wait until the second half of first year to begin research. It's best to get the lay of the land when starting out. You need to figure out how to study and how to manage the vast amounts of material along with the necessary hands-on experiences. Getting organized for research in the summer after first year is probably the best time for a reasonable project.

If summer research is your goal, investigate any structured programs your medical school may have for paid or unpaid summer research options. These are great programs because they often have ready-made mentors and a structured time course for the research to progress.

Investigate any structured programs your medical school may have for paid or unpaid summer research options.

If there's no such program at your school, you can speak to an upper-level student who may know faculty who are good mentors. If upper-level students are applying to the specialty you are interested in, they are perfect people to ask about research mentors.

Contacting a Mentor and Time Management for Research

Once you identify a mentor, you need to figure out the best way to reach them. At our medical school, faculty are very responsive, but that's not always the case. That means you must walk the thin line between being persistent and being a pest. First, try emailing with a follow-up message after approximately one week. If that's not effective, it might be a good idea to find an administrative assistant or research director for the mentor in question. If that doesn't work, it is likely time to pick a new mentor.

Once you get a mentor to agree to do a project with you, the next part of the plan is to figure out how the topic and project are going to progress. Does the mentor have projects that are already underway that you will join? Do they have a separate project for you that will be an offshoot of their research? Is the project clinical or basic science? Basic science projects are usually quite long and involved, so you may wish to ask if your portion of the project can be a poster or abstract for a meeting. Of course, do this after the full discussion of the project, since you don't want to seem ungrateful. If there are other students or residents on the project, it can be a good idea to ask how likely it is that you will be first author on the project. Even if you aren't first author, do your best work, as it may lead to more projects, a great letter of reference, and/or a residency spot.

If you have a difficult time working on research while trying to study for your regular courses, it might be best to utilize a month-long elective early in your fourth year of medical school to complete a research month. This could be too late in the game for some schools, but for others, it's a great time to complete projects after you've had enough medical training to understand how to approach medical questions more aggressively.

One student from my medical school completed a project with every faculty member in the dermatology department starting in his second year of medical school. By the time he was a fourth-year medical student, he had the curriculum vitae of someone who had taken a year off to do research. He was focused, versatile, and easy to work with. That is what you need to be. He also researched all the data, returned an outline quickly, and was a great writer. This is a chance to show how effective you can be on a research project.

This young man matched in dermatology, and it was clear that his work and work ethic helped him get there.

What Not to Do When It Comes to Mentors

There are some mentors who are not the most supportive. If there are students who point out faculty who are not favorites of early researchers, don't attempt to work with them. It's unlikely that you will be the student to change a faculty member's ways. Some faculty members are better with advanced researchers, and there are some who are more focused on their own careers. There are few faculty members who have questionable research ethics, but they do exist. Don't be a part of a fateful tale of someone who works hard on a research project only to be put very low on an author list or left off altogether.

I've also had students and residents who pled with me to mentor them on a project. Once I agreed and discussed what I expected and shared the details of the project, several of them ghosted me. This is very annoying to everyone. Faculty members have no idea if you are going to complete the project or if something happened to you. If you cannot complete the project, just say so. This is much better than just pretending you never started the project in the first place.

This happened to me once. One resident from another program worked with me to help organize a project. She was visiting for one month and was able to do a bit of work on the project. She promised she would complete the project after she left. I contacted her several times to see if she'd made any progress. She rarely answered me, and when she did, she didn't have any updates about the research. An entire year later, a resident from the same program came to work with me and asked about a project. I told her about the project the other resident had started, and the new visiting resident completed the research and published it. To be inclusive, I contacted the first resident to review the work and sign the authorship papers as second author. (At this point, I could have easily cut her out of the project since the idea was mine, her contributions were small, and she was incommunicado for one year.) While I thought I was being nice, the first resident was horrified that I let someone else work on the project and that she was being relegated to second author. This is unrealistic behavior, so don't act like this if you cannot complete a project.

I've had several students work on projects up to the point that they begin their internship. The timing of this means that they had already matched into dermatology by the time the project was coming to an end. By this point, the student has graduated and achieved what they hoped and are now in one of the busiest years of their life. That means I'm left holding the bag for completing the project and submitting it for publication—with all the editorial changes that can occur. It is no secret that my least favorite part of research is submitting projects and completing editorial changes, so when I must do this for a student project, it's very exasperating.

You may think it doesn't matter what happens as long as you match, but you never know when you are going to need a letter of recommendation or a job, so it is best not to start your career by ghosting your research preceptor. Also, dermatology is a very small community, and everyone knows everyone, so don't burn your bridges. If you take on the work, you need to see it through, even if you

It is best not to start your career by ghosting your research preceptor.

must prioritize the research over other things in internship year. Remember that research always takes longer than you think it will, and you need to be the person who moves your project forward.

> You need to be the person who moves your project forward.

Number of Projects and Gap Years

So how many research projects will you need to complete to be competitive? There's no magic number. If you have a huge research paper accepted in a major journal, that may be all you really need. If you have three to four peer-reviewed publications, that's enough for most programs. The most important thing is that you do the work, understand the work, and talk about the work with ease. Even if your work was only published as a poster or abstract at a meeting, that can be just right. Often, it takes time to get a full paper published, so don't sweat the numbers. If a program counts the number of articles of an applicant as most important and you don't have a large number of articles, perhaps you and this program aren't a good fit.

What about the ever-popular gap year for research? This is getting more and more common in dermatology. This year can be taken between your third and fourth year of medical school or after an internship if a match in the specialty didn't occur. This year is best for those who really want to get more exposure to research because they would like research to be a part of their ultimate career or those who haven't had enough exposure to dermatology to have a competitive application (or if there are other weak aspects of their applications). If you can find a research year that pays for your time, that is best. Try not to go into debt while completing a research year.

You'll gain many things beyond the research itself. You can get clinical experience with your mentor or others in the department where you work. You can see how the residents work and progress, and you can have time to volunteer and/or show leadership. Just don't assume that this year is going to be all you need. You will need to be an amazing fellow or the year will be a waste, so don't get the year and just try to sail through it. Make your mark so that your department sees that they can't pass up an opportunity to have you as a resident in their program.

The last thing to remember is that research can truly move the specialty forward, so don't lose sight of this. It may be mostly about what you need to do for your application, but it is also about how you can help your mentor move their research and disseminate this information to other dermatologists and patients who need medical help.

11

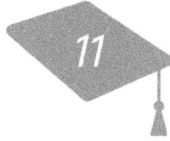

Writing the Best Personal Statement

The personal statement isn't the most important part of the residency application, but it can help the residency get a better idea of who you are. I have read amazing personal statements that didn't lead to an interview, but if the application is top notch, the personal statement can boost your chances of an interview just a bit.

Before writing the statement, think about the message you want to give the residency program. This is a message that no other part of your application can tell. Thus, the statement isn't a recapitulation of what's already listed in your application.

The other important goal of the statement is to let the residency program know why they should hire you for the job of resident. In your past, as a high school student applying to college or as a college student applying to medical school, you were applying for one position out of at least one hundred or more spots at any given school. In most competitive residencies, you are now applying for one position out of approximately four or six in any given program.

That means that you need to make a personal connection—one that is memorable in a single page.

Pitfalls and Fixes

One of the biggest pitfalls I see in personal statements is that the statement is too long. When programs have over five hundred applications to review, long personal statements are overwhelming and stressful to read. Keep the statement to one page. Trimming your statement is a good way to make sure your thoughts are concise and specific to the task.

> Long personal statements are overwhelming and stressful to read. Keep the statement to one page.

I have read two- and three-page treatises on all the skin conditions of everyone in the applicant's family. You don't have to tell us about these kinds of things because we already know that a lot of people have skin conditions. If there is one particular skin disease (in one person) that was important in piquing your interest in dermatology, that would be fine to mention, but only for two or three sentences at most.

Also, don't try to make the statement too dramatic. This is not the time to work on your novel-writing skills. Well-written does not mean trying to emulate Jane Austen or William Shakespeare. Too much flowery writing can overshadow your medical excellence.

Another pitfall is defining dermatology in your statement. We all know that the specialty is visual and that it affects people of all ages, races, and ethnicities, since we are all practicing dermatologists. Every time the applicant committee reads this, they roll their eyes and the application loses points. You'll have to be more creative in convincing us why you like the specialty of dermatology and why you're best for the job.

Also, don't make the statement too short. If you only have one or two paragraphs on the page, it seems like you don't really have much to say about the specialty or that you're lazy. So, do fill the page at least three-quarters full.

Don't name drop. It's great if you have worked with a dermatology star, but their accolades don't make *you* a star. You need to convince us why you're worthy and deserve a spot in our residency.

I have seen a few statements that speak ill of the applicant's previous places of study. Even if you haven't had a stellar experience at your college or medical school, don't air the specifics of that dirty laundry in a personal statement. Find something positive about your previous educational experiences or simply say little about it. Less is more in this situation.

Don't write a poem for your personal statement unless your poetry has won major awards, and maybe not even then. Believe it or not, there are a few applicants who have done this. I have even seen a haiku for a personal statement. There is a rare person who should do this, so it would be best not to try it.

Finally, I never thought I would say this, but don't harp on the fact that you are a person of color and that there is a need for more people with skin of color in dermatology. Those of us who care about this know it already, and those who don't care also don't want to hear it. You can mention something about interest in studying the topic of skin of color dermatology, but just being a person of color does not make you a fantastic candidate. That is something you will need to show in your actions and accomplishments.

What You Should Include

Okay, so now you know what not to include in the statement, but what *should* you include to really wow the applicant review committee? You can make the most of this statement by showing the committee why you are right for the position. You can mention why you like the specialty (remember, no definitions), but that should be minimal. We know why dermatology is great. We need to know what *you* have done that makes you a good fit for the specialty and for our program. What will you bring to our program that makes you hard to pass up?

We want to see how your leadership was critical to a committee or organization in medical school. It's fine if you did lots of leadership work in college, but we want to see what you have accomplished more currently. This leadership can be inside or outside medical school, but it just needs to show a pattern of taking on responsibility while dealing with the rigor of medical school. The other thing you need to show is what traits and experiences will make you the best dermatology resident. This is your chance to take one or two of the research studies that you worked on and talk about your pivotal role in the project.

Show what traits and experiences will make you the best dermatology resident.

Try to do a bit of a personal assessment when you write your statement. What can you do or bring that is very important or helpful in residency? Do you have more pediatric experience than the usual applicant? Do you have experience of practicing medicine or a rotation in another country? Did you work in a developing country at some time in your life? Are you a writer or singer? Do you do something particularly unusual for your well-being? Anything that helps you stand out in a positive way can be helpful.

Some people will talk about a specific case they observed in clinic or in the hospital. That is fine if you have something that you did as part of the case that was pivotal. No one on the applicant committee wants to hear about a case just for the heck of it. We see enough cases every day.

Finally, you can also include distance traveled if you have such a story and wish to share. You shouldn't feel compelled to tell your deepest, darkest secrets or things that are painful for you to discuss. But, for example, if you don't have a dermatology department at your medical school, it can be helpful to discuss how you navigated getting dermatology experience without the help of a home department. Also, if you have immigrated to this country or have an uncommon background, these can all be interesting points to share.

There is no right answer about what to discuss when it comes to your ethnicity or race, but there is a trend to block demographic information about applicants, which means that there is no way for the various programs to know if you are an URiM applicant. If this is something that is important for you to convey, then it may be something that you want to weave into your personal statement. It should be woven in such a way that you are telling a story that is relevant to your application to dermatology rather than just stating your race/ethnicity as a matter of course.

115

The Best Personal Statements

It is safe to say that every residency program may look for different things in a personal statement, but we can all agree that some are simply stellar. One particularly good example is a statement where a student started with a story about her own journey through a serious medical illness. She was clear about what happened to her, how she recovered, and how that recovery had changed her outlook and given her the resiliency to pursue dermatology. She was able to speak about a difficult time in her life but presented it in a way that made her seem better than the average candidate and a great person for the job.

Another great personal statement was one that described how the applicant was a teenage mother but was able to complete high school to get a scholarship and ultimately go to medical school. This could have been a harrowing story, but it was written in a very uplifting way and left me, the reader, feeling that this applicant was something special.

Not everyone is going to have a devastating life event to discuss. Some of the best statements are those that discuss the journey of becoming a solid person, medical student, athlete, or researcher. All these stories have a common thread: a description of their character and intrinsic qualities. These show what can be expected from the applicant when they get here. They provide a glimpse into how you've become the person you are and what you will accomplish because of your past experiences.

Final Thoughts on the Statement

Remember to have at least three people read your statement before you upload it to your application. I recommend having your parents or someone your parents' age, someone in your medical school class who isn't applying to dermatology, and perhaps a mentor who knows what a dermatology personal statement should look like. Each of these people can give valuable feedback. Even if you decide not to take their advice, at least you will know how folks in these different arenas interpret what you have written. Just make sure to write early enough to give your readers time to make edits and comments.

> Have at least three people read your statement before you upload it to your application.

Check for typos. This is a no-brainer, but sometimes students don't do this.

I recommend not using artificial intelligence to write your statement. Recently, when we included an extra bonus question on our application, two applicants had exactly the same answers. People notice similarities between different essays, so try to make this statement your own work.

Last, have a bit of fun writing about yourself. It is not often you get to do this *and* have it help you move to the next level of your career.

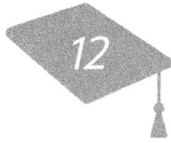

LETTERS OF RECOMMENDATION

NOW THAT MOST MEDICAL SCHOOLS ARE PASS/FAIL FOR THE first two years and there are few ranking systems, it becomes very difficult to distinguish between applicants when reviewing applications. The few things that can really help highlight a great applicant are excellence in strong research, leadership, volunteerism, and letters of recommendation. The letters of recommendation tell the programs who you are and how you interacted with the faculty dermatologists on rotation or with research. They also give an estimation of how you stack up against current and past applicants in terms of your work ethic, knowledge, and morals. Thus, you need to ask the right people the right questions to get letters that best represent your work and personality.

Who Should Be Writing Your Letters

There's some debate about who should write letters of recommendation. I believe that you should submit at least three letters, four if possible, on the final application. You should have at least two letters from dermatology faculty members who are well acquainted with your personality as well as your clinical/research experience and prowess. These letter writers should be mid-career to senior (if you have that option), because this gives you a writer with experience and knowledge about how to present you as competitive with others. Early career faculty are fine as well if those are the people who know you best. Always go with those who know you best rather than those who may be well known in the field but have minimal knowledge of who you are and what you've accomplished.

> You should submit at least three letters, four if possible, on the final application.

Letters from those who don't know you show poorly in the application. It's easy to spot them because they just give a rundown of your CV and very little personal information. By all means, if you have a well-known physician with whom you have worked extensively, they can be a great letter writer. I had one candidate submit a letter from the world-renowned physician and author, Abraham Verghese, because he had worked closely with the student in a longitudinal fashion and could comment on the student's path and developmental progress over the course of medical school. That was pretty cool to read and a great letter for the applicant as well.

The third letter can be from a physician from another discipline, like internal medicine, pediatrics, or a subspecialty of internal medicine. I recommend these particular areas of medicine because letters from faculty in surgical disciplines (with the exception of dermatologic surgery) tend to be more about surgical abilities than commitment to outpatient medicine and diagnostic abilities. Another touchy subject is the fact that students who stress the surgical component of dermatology may be viewed as only wanting to go into our specialty to ultimately practice Mohs surgery, which can be considered a red flag for an applicant, suggesting they won't give their all to the medical and pathology components of the residency. It is no secret that Mohs surgeons do well financially and typically have a higher income than medical dermatologists, but if you associate yourself with this too early, you may not be viewed as a well-rounded applicant. There is nothing wrong with enjoying procedures, but that should only be a part of what is highlighted in your letters. You do not want to be perceived as viewing dermatology as "plastic surgery–lite" or "otolaryngology-lite."

The best option for the third letter is someone in your medical school who knows you in a longitudinal way. This is important because this letter writer will have a perspective of you as a whole person. It could be an advisor or someone who was a research mentor early in medical school or even a section director for a course in which you particularly excelled. This is actually something to consider early in your time in medical school. Having an early mentoring relationship will definitely help you overall and will give you the opportunity to ask that mentor for a letter later in the relationship.

> Having an early mentoring relationship will give you the opportunity to ask that mentor for a letter later in the relationship.

The fourth letter is really a toss-up. It can be another derm letter if you're lucky enough to have another person in the specialty who knows you well. It can also be from someone with whom you've worked on research, even if not dermatologic research. I have read a number of excellent letters that were written by non-derm investigators with whom the applicant worked in a summer off from medical school or continued to work with during the school year.

What Not to Use as a Letter of Recommendation

Each year, there are few applicants who do not have dermatology departments at their medical school, and they include letters of recommendation from pure private practice dermatologists. This is a problem because these individuals often do not have the longitudinal experience with other medical students that would give them the ability to discern who is truly an amazing applicant versus a smart medical student who catches on fast to computer issues. But there are some very academic dermatologists who are in private practice. They may teach students and residents on a regular basis, perform research, and present nationally on specialty areas of dermatology. This type of person is fine as a letter writer.

Another letter type that we occasionally see is the hometown dermatologist who, again, has no exposure to a breadth of students. It is nice that they have seen you grow up, but we can't use this kind of letter, so don't include it. Also don't get your parents' dermatology friend to write you a letter. They are usually short, terse, and not substantive.

Finally, do not use the composite letter from the Internal Medicine rotation, where many different residents and faculty members discuss your work on that rotation. It rarely gives insight into your dermatology abilities and is just difficult to read—and

> Don't get your parents' dermatology friend to write you a letter.

overall, not helpful. When I see this letter in an application, it sends the message that this applicant is lazy and doesn't want to take the time to ask someone for a specific letter, or that the applicant is clueless on what this composite letter actually looks like. Either way, it's not a good idea to include it. Take these letters very seriously and give thought to who will write them and how well they can represent you as the whole package to a residency program.

> Take these letters very seriously and give thought to who will write them.

Requesting a Letter of Recommendation

Approaching faculty members for letters of recommendation is a bit of an art. If you are lucky enough to have faculty members offer to write you a letter of recommendation, that's great! Make sure to consider these individuals as letter writers if they fulfill the appropriate criteria for the requirements of the letter. Be careful not to ask a famous physician to write you a letter just because of who they are if they don't know you well.

Asking for letters while on away rotation is a delicate matter. It would be best to complete at least two weeks of the rotation and make sure to have worked several times with whomever you ask.

When to ask for a letter is important as well. I prefer that students ask me to write letters at a time when I am not in the middle of something else. It can be a scheduled time that the student gets on my calendar, or it can be when a student asks before the start of clinic or after clinic. That allows for more than a cursory conversation.

Once this time is scheduled, make sure to update and bring your current CV and your personal statement (if completed) for the faculty member if they agree to writing your letter. This will help them see other things that you have done that they may not know about, allowing them to comment on these achievements along with their observations of you.

Applicants asking for letters of support should ask if the potential letter writer would be able to write them a *strong* letter of recommendation, with emphasis on the "strong." Most people will be honest with you about whether they feel comfortable writing a strong letter, but others won't, and that's a chance you will have to take. However, you can do a bit of research from students who are ahead of you and current residents in the department about who writes great letters.

> Ask if the potential letter writer would be able to write you a STRONG letter of recommendation, with emphasis on the "strong."

What you don't want is someone who agrees to write you a letter even though they're not necessarily excited about it. Letters from these letter writers are usually very brief and terse and not at all what you really want—which is someone who says that you walk on water. Frankly, you need people who are in your corner to go big on the letter and not give a trite discussion of your punctuality and good comments in clinic. You really want someone to sing your praises. I read a letter of recommendation some years ago that was approximately five lines long and not very complimentary to the applicant. I had met this applicant through family connections previously, and I did break confidence to let her know this letter was part of her application. She had absolutely no idea that he had written such a letter. So be careful when you select your letter writer and don't go to taciturn people who don't know you well. Go to your cheerleader to get the best letter you can get.

13

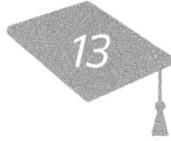

How to Prepare for the Interview

THE INTERVIEW FOR RESIDENCY IS TOWARD THE END OF THE line in the entire application process for dermatology, but it can make or break your acceptance into a program. With thirty years of experience as an academic dermatologist, twelve years as a program director, and eleven years as a chair, I can assure you that I have seen hundreds of ways that make or break a residency interview. We take the interviews very seriously. We have to spend three years with residents, and we don't want to spend that time with someone who doesn't have an ethical code or values that we hold in high esteem at our program.

Preparing for the interview can be challenging because it's the culmination of a lot of work, but with only eight to twelve minutes of face time with the program. There may be more time with the residents if the program has a resident applicant information session. The biggest change in the interview process over the last few years has been the conversion from in-person interviews to virtual interviews. As time moves on, it is likely that there will be a swing of the pendulum back to more in-person interviews, so I'll discuss both.

Before the Interview

Before the interview, you need to make sure you complete several tasks. The first task is to review everything you put on your curriculum vitae (CV). If you put it on your CV, it is fair game for the interviewers to ask about.

Review everything you put on your CV. If you put it on your CV, it is fair game for the interviewers to ask about.

It's disappointing to me when I ask about research on an applicant's CV and their response is that they do not know the outcome because they were only involved for a short time. You need to make it your business to know what happened if you list it—or simply do not list it. Particularly, if you write a paper on a topic, you need to understand the results and be able to discuss every aspect of the research presented. Again, it is a bad look when you are confused about the data or have a hard time explaining recruitment of patients. Not only should you be clear on the research process, but you also need to be able to explain it in a few short sentences. The interview is short, and you don't want to take the whole interview answering one question. This means you need to practice a brief, comprehensive answer about each research, committee, and volunteer experience you list.

Handling Gaps in Your Educational Years

If there are gaps in your education, you also need to be able discuss how you spent your time during those gaps. If you have had medical issues or family responsibilities causing your time away from school, that's fine to discuss, but don't tell all parts of your personal information. That will just be too much. Practice a succinct way to explain these times that is hopeful and not depressing, even if the reason for the break was not a happy one.

> Practice a succinct way to explain gaps that is hopeful and not depressing.

I have interviewed several applicants who have had personal illness that required months off during medical school, but their explanations showed resilience and confidence. Some applicants may have lost a parent or other family member, and there's no way to spin that as a positive, but it can also show that you understand how to weather a sad and devastating loss. Others may need to take time off to have children, which is very acceptable. Simply be matter of fact if this was your decision. If there are programs who don't like this, that is short-sighted and inappropriate but may be their prerogative. How you decide to handle this is a personal decision, but these are just some ideas to consider.

How to Dress for the Interview

You also need to consider what you will wear during your interview. This may be easy for most applicants, but give some thought to how your suit or outfit looks. Is it dated? Does it still fit properly? How will it travel?

Also, make sure you always keep the outfit with you when you travel. I had one applicant who came to his interview wearing jeans and a zip hoodie. He told us that his luggage was lost after he checked it—and that this was the third time this had happened. That let me know that he did not think ahead and perhaps was low on common sense. I knew immediately that he wasn't going to be a good fit for our program. I enjoyed speaking with him, but it was a no-go for ranking him. If you have an important interview, bring your luggage as carry-on rather than checked luggage.

For those who wear makeup, a more conservative look is best for interviews. This is not the time to try out the latest fads in dark colors around your eyes or shocking pink lipstick. Try for a toned-down version of your usual makeup and make sure your lighting (if virtual) is appropriate for the makeup you choose.

If you're interviewing virtually, spend a bit of time to design a nice background for your interview. Make sure you have a good light source so you are visible to the interviewers. If you have your own artwork or art collection, this can be a nice conversation starter. If you're not into art or design, you should still work on having a pleasant background with a bit of interest for your interviewers to look at. A blank wall can make you look like you're in prison, so try not to have that. Make sure you wear what you would wear in an in-person interview. Also, make sure your computer and internet connections are working well. It is tedious spending the entire interview telling the applicant that we can't hear them. It uses your time and is distracting. It may also mean that you will be out of the running for the residency position since your interview is truncated.

Practice Makes Perfect

Once you have your outfit selected and your background in place, it is a good idea to have a practice interview or two prior to the actual day. There are several groups that provide practice interview experiences for residency applicants, including the National Medical Association (NMA) dermatology section. Your own school may provide this, or you may be able to schedule a session with your mentor. This will not take long, since interviews are approximately eight to ten minutes. Allow for fifteen minutes of feedback after the practice interview, and everything can be completed in thirty minutes or less.

Prior to the interview, you should also look up the website of the department. Be familiar with the chair, the program director, and perhaps a bit about the city where the residency program is located. If you have time to look up the faculty, that can be helpful as well. This can help give you questions that pertain to certain faculty members based on your interests.

Contacting the Program for Questions

Don't call the residency program coordinators with questions that are answered in the paperwork they already sent. It's fine to clarify if things are not clearly outlined, but fully read the information sent before you call. It makes you look a bit needy if you ask a lot of questions that are already discussed in your packet, and you should be aware that the coordinators do share the phone and email etiquette of the applicants with the program director when there are unusual requests or frequent questions.

We had one applicant call to ask if her fiancé (who did not receive an interview from our program) could come along for a practice interview. We of course told her no. That was strike one. Then she called on the day of the interview stating that she missed her flight and wanted to reschedule at a time that was not previously offered. We don't play into those kinds of requests, so she was immediately disqualified for ranking. Perhaps she was not particularly interested in our program anyway, so that is okay for her, but don't do this at any program you are still considering for ranking. I found out later that this same applicant made similar requests at another program—they made efforts to set up a whole new time for her to meet multiple faculty members, and she never showed up. The hint here is that programs talk about applicant outliers. Remember that dermatology is a small world and crazy stories about you might be shared.

The Day of the Interview

When the interview day comes, in-person interviews will require much more preparation. Make sure that you arrive on the correct day. Many years ago, we had an applicant come on the wrong interview day, but we chose to interview him anyway. That should have been a huge red flag to us, but we ultimately matched this person to our residency and found him to have major issues with time management among other things. This required a significant amount of my time to help him develop tools to get organized and be prepared for life as a dermatologist. We won't make this error in judgment again, so be careful with dates and times. You need to arrive early for the day so that the introductory process can start on time. Also, there are often tours that begin soon after the start of the day, as it is customary to split the interview group into two groups with one group going on a tour first and the second group beginning the interviews.

The Entire Day Is Your Interview

While at the interview, your behavior is on view from the time you walk into the department until the time you leave. You might even consider that any contact you have with the department will be noticed, and that includes with staff, residents, and faculty. That means that you should assume anything that you say or do with other applicants while not in the actual interviews is noted by the program coordinators who are planning the day, and this information is shared with the faculty at some point before ranking. One applicant decided to give his opinion of how people who do not go to college are not bright enough to sit on juries for trials. We had no idea why he was discussing this topic, but the program coordinators overheard his comments, and they were not well-received by either the coordinators or the rest of the faculty once we found out.

133

There are simply some topics that are not appropriate to discuss on the day of the interview, whether it's in the interview or not. I have had applicants share a photo album of more than 20 photos of their cats and another try to work through very complicated issues of gender preference in their short 8–10 minutes. Even if your interviewer seems down-to-earth and kind, this is not the time to get in a psychology session while interviewing. A rule of thumb is: don't share anything during your interview that would be best shared with your psychiatrist.

It should go without saying that you should not use the interview time to work on getting dates with other applicants. One applicant tried to ask another applicant out on a date during downtime on the interview day. Again, this was overheard by our residency coordinators. He was quickly relegated to the bottom of our rank list. Also, please use the restroom before leaving on tour. This should be common sense for someone who is an adult, but we had a male applicant who did not go to the restroom prior to the offsite bus tour of the city and had to stop the bus to go to the bathroom in the bushes on the side of the road. This did not go over well with the other applicants or the rest of the faculty when we found out. When I asked him about what happened, he told me that he had more coffee than he usually drinks and did not realize he would need to go to the restroom so soon. I will just tell you that you need to have more foresight than that as a physician, so this person was a no-go for us. Overall, he was a nice guy and had done a good amount of research, but that one thing gave us a reason to take him off our rank list. Remember, if you make it to the interview, you have a good shot at matching. One small thing can take you off the list, so make sure you avoid these missteps.

Fielding Questions During the Interview

There's often a part of the interview where interviewers ask about your research, how you're spending your time during the month of your interview, or something about your CV. Be prepared for questions that may be difficult to answer or even inappropriate. It's fine to consider your words for a few seconds before you answer. When you're asked about what you are doing during the time of the interview, please talk about something that is reasonably academic. We realize that interviews come at a time when many fourth-year medical students have a lighter schedule than during the rest of medical school, but don't allow yourself to seem like a slacker.

> It's fine to consider your words for a few seconds before you answer.

One applicant who was asked this question answered that he was making sure that he kept up his perfect record of watching every show and movie on Netflix. To some, that may be a great achievement, but we didn't see it as such. Another applicant seemed to think I was one of her contemporaries when I asked what she was doing during the last few months of medical school. She said, "Girrrl, you know I am chilling and hanging out with my friends in my hometown." I even tried to give her a chance to redeem herself by asking about if she was doing research or rotations while she was there, and she again reiterated how she was finished with her medical school obligations and wasn't doing anything related to medicine. That's not the sentiment I wanted to hear.

Medicine doesn't have to fill every part of your life, but you only get exposure to that level of medical education once in your life, and I would much rather rank someone for residency who knows how to take advantage of this than someone who is only focused on fun. That last applicant did not match into any residency and contacted me about what she could have done differently. I absolutely let her know that she should have seen the interview as a gift and that she should have done everything she could to make sure she remained professional rather than being overly familiar with me and talking only about relaxation.

> When your interviewer asks if you have any questions, it is best if you have at least one question in queue.

When your interviewer asks if you have any questions, it is best if you have at least one question in queue. Even if you have asked questions throughout the day and are tired, have a few things to ask about. It is a bit deflating when an interviewer asks if you have questions, and you say that you don't really have anything.

Interacting with the Current Program Residents

If you are interviewing in person, there's usually a pre-interview dinner with the residents the night before. If you seem bored during that dinner, rest assured, the faculty will hear about it, so try to get interested in conversation with the residents. Also, this should go without saying, but don't drink too much. We have several stories about those who overindulge. This is not a good look.

As virtual interviews became popular, online residency meet and greets with the applicants and the residency group have become common as well. This is usually scheduled the night before the actual interviews or on the same day, either before or after the interviews with faculty. These meetings are usually informal with a brief presentation and an opportunity for the applicants to ask questions of the current residents in a program. If you have travel or other important duties during this meeting, it's not the end of the world to miss it, but it can be helpful in determining if the residents are happy or if they feel there are gaps in the training they're receiving. If you attend this meeting, make sure to pay attention. Residents have been able to see reflections of some applicants' screens while they're shopping on Amazon or checking Instagram. If you must do these things, just don't attend, because anyone the residents report as doing this will be quickly dropped off our rank list.

After the Interview

Many applicants feel obligated to send thank you notes after residency interviews, but most, if not all, residency programs would rather *not* receive emails or notes from the fifty or more applicants that they interview. If there is a particular thing that requires follow up, such as a discussion about a paper that you were to send or a book recommendation you were asked to give, that's fine. It's too much to thank every person with whom you interview. If you must send a note, it's best to send it only to the program director or the program coordinator for them to distribute to others as they see fit.

> Most, if not all, residency programs would rather *not* receive thank you emails or notes from the 50 or more applicants that they interview.

When the time comes for your final rank list submission for residency, you can certainly email the program director your top programs to let them know they are at the top of your list. Don't expect the program director to discuss the program rankings, since this is against the Matching Program rules, but they can note this as they build their list. Try to figure out your rank list early, so you can contact the program before they submit their own list.

Last but not least, *relax* when it comes to your interview. You are the best authority on you, and you just have to practice putting your best foot forward.

14

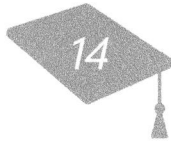

Failure Is Not Fatal

One of the worst feelings in the world is when you find out that something you worked hard to learn and master turns out to be a failure. Whether it's a paper, a final exam, a board exam, or a course—your stomach drops, your face heats up, and your stress hormones start the fight or flight response. It is a feeling we've all had at one time or another, and it's not one that we look forward to.

When this stress happens, it can feel like there's no way out; doom and gloom can set in. As the doom starts to descend, you need to shake it off and jump into action. It may feel good to go home and eat a pint of ice cream while you pout (and you can do this), but don't stop there. Tell a true friend about the failure to get it off your chest. Then start planning the steps to rectify the issue.

My Medical School Failure

I personally felt this when I failed the cardiology block of our pathophysiology course in medical school. I had never failed any class or major test in the past, so it was a gut punch when I received this failure after studying so hard. It took some time to process, but as I examined what happened to cause it, I realized that I didn't use a strategic plan to study.

I had studied hard and a lot, but not in an organized way. The lack of organization had me flailing around, trying to study the notes from class as well as readings from our text without a deep understanding of the material. I believe some of this lack of organization was due to the volume of material that had to be studied for several tests taking place each day for three days in a row. Another issue was that I tended to skim the surface of materials as a learned poor study habit.

I had to look internally and face the things I needed to change. Then I needed to work on how to remediate this horrible misstep. I called the Student Affairs Diversity counselor, and she had no suggestions. Apparently four students failed this test (which should have told them that this wasn't the best test in the first place, but I digress), and this would be a matter for one of the deans to determine. We were all good students up to that point, and we represented ourselves well in discussions with this dean. The dean first proposed that the four of us would enter into our clinical rotations one month late and take a makeup exam to determine if we could start the clinical rotations at all. We didn't see why we needed to be punished by not being allowed to enter clinical rotations. It would have been embarrassing for us and not necessary for remediation. We were able to advocate for a remediation exam and recommended that we just miss the first day of orientation for the start of rotations while we took the exam. We were able to use the winter break to study, and we all used it wisely and passed. None of us had a major shift to our educational journey; we moved forward with our class.

Not All Leaders Can Help When Failure Occurs

In summary, we had a stressful failure that seemed like the end of the world at first. When I turned to someone in a leadership role, and she was of no help, it was another blow. Luckily, I had several close friends in whom I could confide and a supportive family who helped me through the worst of it.

The school should have had a plan in place for any eventuation so the dean wouldn't have to step in to decide. Now, there are usually well-worked-out considerations when there is a failure of any kind in medical school, so that takes away the guesswork. It also makes it more fair for the student, and it's supportive rather than punitive. However, that doesn't mean that every person is going to be supportive, so you still must get mentors who will help support and advise you.

> Get mentors who will help support and advise you through both success and failure.

What Not to Do When Faced with Failure

One cautionary tale about failure was exemplified by one of my student mentees. I had a student who started medical school sure that dermatology was her career choice. She came to meet with me just after the beginning of her first year and discussed how she discovered dermatology while working in a plastic surgery office as a medical assistant between college and medical school. She had a sparkle in her eye and a sparkly personality to go with it. She kept in touch with me over her first year and planned an extended research time with me. During that research time, she was a joy to work with, and she meshed well with our residents and faculty. I figured she would be a sure thing when it came time to match into residency. Unfortunately, before she could get to that point, she fell off the radar. This was a while ago, and I was not as thorough a mentor. I did reach out a few times, but I assumed she was busy.

I hadn't heard from this student for over a year when she finally made an appointment for us to meet. During this meeting, she explained that she had not contacted me because she had failed Step 1 of the boards. She was both devastated and embarrassed. She explained that she had been concerned about a serious medical diagnosis she had just received and was going through testing related to this diagnosis. She spoke to a leader in the medical school who advised her that if she could walk, she needed to go and take the test. So she did just that. It was no surprise that she did poorly, as she couldn't concentrate on studying or the exam during that trying time in her life. Once that happened, she explained she didn't know who to contact or what to do.

After we spoke, the student took a short leave of absence to work on her health issue, which resolved and was not ultimately a serious concern. Her family was not particularly supportive, and she lost complete faith in her abilities. Ultimately, she did return to her clinical rotations and was supposed to make plans to retake the board exam. I assumed things were progressing as we had discussed and tried to contact her. I did not receive a response and found out through a vice dean in the medical school that the student never took the exam again and had left medical school. She was not answering the calls of anyone at the medical center.

To this day, I haven't heard a word from this amazing young woman. I think of her often and wonder if there was more I could have done, but the truth of the matter is that she was not ready to accept the mentorship my department offered her. She would have had to meet us halfway by contacting us when she faced her dilemmas, something that did not allow her to accept my help. My hope is that she's doing well wherever she is and that our paths cross again in time.

> Meet your mentors halfway by contacting them when you face dilemmas.

Learning from Failure

Another mentee story illustrates how one can learn from failure. A student from an outside medical school contacted me about coming to visit for a mentorship using a grant from a national society. I was happy to have her visit because she didn't have a dermatology department at her medical school. She was a great rotator. She was able to shadow me, and we discussed options for her as she moved through the process of a strong medical school performance. We met virtually intermittently, and then she, too, informed me that she failed Step 1 of the boards. She had already recovered and retaken the test and passed. She scheduled the meeting to discuss her options after this recovery, which was exactly where she needed to be.

We are still in process and will have to see what happens, but this kind of comeback after devastation is commendable. And that's all you can ask. She'll likely need to complete a research year if she doesn't have a lucky break with a program where she rotates, but she's open to the work and ready for the challenge.

Not Matching, the Ultimate Failure

Not matching in dermatology the first time is the fate no one wants to face. Even thirty-plus years ago when I was applying to dermatology, when others learned I was applying for dermatology, the next question was always: "What will you do if you don't match?" This question has only become more common when applying to dermatology, as it's even more competitive now than it was back then. Applicants have lots of hoops to jump through. Even some wonderfully prepared students do not match.

So, what do you do if you fail to match? First, you need to go to your support family and friends and get all the emotions out. This will be a disappointment, but it is one you can get past.

After you lick your wounds and recover, you must take stock of your application and how competitive it truly was. Talk with your dean of medical students, your mentor, and the dermatology program director at your institution if there is one. If applying to derm was a last-minute idea and if your application did not have the requisite parts (research, letters of recommendation, volunteerism, mentorship, interviews) set up for success, then you'll need to meet with your mentor to see what needs to be addressed. If you received a good number of interviews, it might be helpful to ask one or two of the program directors from the interviewing programs how you could have done better or for any other constructive advice they may have.

If everything was complete in the application and you are ready for more hard work, there are several ways to proceed. I usually recommend completing an internship even if you don't match in dermatology because there are always a few residency spots that appear after the match or during the following year, and you'll only be prepared to take advantage of them if you have completed your internship. This isn't a sure thing, but if your mentor can tell you when these spots become available, it can be a way to get into derm without having to plan a year off between internship and residency.

Lately, some students have been extending medical school an extra year with research or an additional degree, and that has worked for some. Other students will complete an internship, then obtain a research position afterward. Either way, the idea is to pick a mentor for the research year or gap year that will enrich your experience rather than just utilize you for their own research. Certainly, getting the research completed is important, but not to the extent that you only have time for research. The best research years will also offer time to shadow or work in clinics, attend conferences, and meet the residents.

It may take more than one year to match after an unsuccessful attempt since some programs do not interview reapplicants, but many others do. Keep the faith and follow the guidelines set out in the previous sections to be the best you can be in the match.

The moral of the story is that failure is not fatal. It can hurt, it can be surreal, it can be devastating, but in the end, it is not fatal unless you allow it to be. The best applicants figure out how to solve the issue and come back to continue to achieve. Plans may have to change, but you will be successful as you move through your career, even if on a different trajectory.

> Failure is not fatal unless you allow it to be.

15

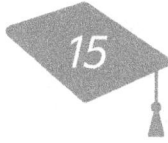

You Matched! Now What?

WHEN ALL YOUR HARD WORK PAYS OFF AND YOU GET INTO your beloved specialty of choice, now what do you do? After the celebration and the much-needed sleep after that, what's next?

What's next is that you don't stop working hard. Now the work is to focus on how you can make the specialty better. Are you going to be involved in research and add to the literature? Are you going to be an educator, teaching others how to examine, diagnose, and treat patients? Will you be a clinical expert in dermatologic surgery, dermatopathology, or pediatric dermatology? Will you serve your hometown or an underserved community or will you brave the busiest of cities to offer something new to patients?

Whatever you decide to do for work, you can start figuring that out in residency. Use the skill and excellence that got you into residency to make yourself an amazing resident in preparation for life as a dermatologist. Getting into residency is not the end goal. It is just the beginning. I see far too many residents have a "good enough" mentality once they are in residency, just hanging on until residency ends. Don't allow that to happen to you.

There is no doubt that residency is difficult (yes, even in dermatology). Having to learn very complex skin pathology after not seeing any pathology since second year of medical school is always a challenge. The genetics and mechanisms of skin disease are ever more complex, and this must all be learned to understand the treatment of inflammatory and oncologic skin diseases.

One star student mentee of mine went to train at a dermatology program in another part of the country to be near her family. The program was a good one, but she encountered a few rocky times after not doing well on one of the required board exam modules. She was also doing a fair amount of racial equity work in her department and medical center in addition to her work as a resident. The failure on the required test despite her efforts to keep up and do advocacy work just seemed to drain the fire out of her. She did not share what she went through with me until after much time had passed, mainly because she seemed ashamed of showing failure.

The beauty of having mentors is being able to come for advice and support in good and bad times. She managed to work through the issues on her own and with the support of friends, but she was never as fired up about her education or potentially entering an academic career as she had been. It is completely fine that she chose to join a practice rather than an academic department, but I wonder what would have happened if she had come to me for perspective during that time of hardship.

You need to continue to find joy in your practice of medicine even during the intensity of studying. I'm not a fan of residents having to take board exams during their

148

residency training, but that is the reality, so don't let studying for and taking these exams steal your joy for the specialty. Find the cases that excite you and read more on those topics—this is the last time you'll have time to delve into your specialty like this. Design a study to answer a question you have about a disease process. Maybe you can design a quality improvement project around an inefficient clinic process. During the ups and downs of residency, you will continue to need mentors. In fact, you will need mentors for the rest of your career, so keep that in mind when you hit roadblocks or issues that are difficult to work out alone.

You will need mentors for the rest of your career

Each of you were chosen because a spark was seen in the application and/or interview. Make sure to live up to this spark. Don't stop being amazing. Be present, bring it, and after residency, know that you "left it all on the floor like Beyoncé" during your training.

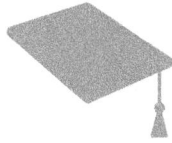

Final Thoughts

I HOPE THIS BOOK WAS HELPFUL FOR YOU. THERE ARE MANY more lessons to learn about being a strong medical student and a good dermatology residency applicant, but I wanted to keep this book relatively short to allow my audience to get through the book and not add to an already busy workload. I have described my journey, which is very specific to me but hopefully gives lessons and guideposts for how to navigate *your* way. I've enjoyed revisiting the interesting stories of students and other learners during my career, and I trust that they'll help you find the correct trajectory for excellence in school and a successful match in dermatology. At the very least, I've offered guidance for developing the technical parts of the application. For students who are URiM, this book offers support for leadership and resilience.

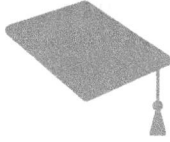

REFERENCES

1. Adam Grant, *Hidden Potential: The Science of Achieving Greater Things,* first large print edition (New York: Random House Large Print, 2023).

2. Verna Meyers, as quoted in Michael Seitchik, "How to Make the Leap from Inclusion to Belonging," *BTS*, May 2020, https://bts.com/insights/how-to-make -the-leap-from-inclusion-to-belonging, accessed October 20, 2024.

3. LaFawn Davis, "How Belonging Differs from Diversity and Inclusion—and Why It Matters," *Indeed for Employers*, September 4, 2021, https://ca.indeed.com /leadershiphub/how-belonging-differs-from-diversity-and-inclusion, accessed October 20, 2024.

4. "Racial and Ethnic Diversity in the United States: 2010 Census and 2020 Census," *United States Census Bureau*, https://www.census.gov/library/visualizations /interactive/racial-and-ethnic-diversity-in-the-united-states-2010-and-2020 -census.html, accessed October 20, 2024.

5. "Table A-12" in "2024 FACTS: Applicants and Matriculants Data," AAMC.org, https://www.aamc.org/media/6046/download, accessed October 21, 2024.

6. Collin M. Costello, et al., "The role of race and ethnicity in the dermatology applicant match process," *Journal of the National Medical Association* 113, 6 (2022): 666–70, doi:10.1016/j.jnma.2021.07.005.

7. Damon Tweedy, *Black Man in a White Coat: A Doctor's Reflections on Race and Medicine* (New York: Picador, 2015).

8. Michelle Weir, "Understanding and Addressing Microaggressions in Medicine," *Dermatologic Clinics* 41, 2 (April 2023): 291–7, doi:10.1016/j.det.2022.08.006.

9. Madeline B. Torres, et al., "Recognizing and Reacting to Microaggressions in Medicine and Surgery," *JAMA Surgery* 154, 9 (July 2019): 868–72, doi:10.1001/ jamasurg.2019.1648.

10. Matthew N. Goldenberg, et al., "ERASE: A New Framework for Faculty to Manage Patient Mistreatment of Trainees," *Academic Psychiatry* 43, 4 (2019): 396–9, doi:10.1007/s40596-018-1011-6.

11. Derald Wing Sue, et al., "Racial Microaggressions in Everyday Life: Implications for Clinical Practice," *American Psychologist* 62, 4 (2007): 271–86, doi:10.1037/0003-066X.62.4.271. And Brittany Feaster, et al., "Microaggressions in Medicine," *Cutis* 107, 5 (May 2021):235–7, doi:10.12788/cutis.0249.

12. Carmine Gallo, *Talk Like TED: The 9 Public Speaking Secrets of the World's Top Minds* (London: Pan Macmillan UK, 2014).

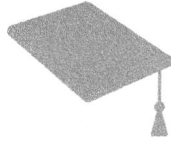

ACKNOWLEDGMENTS

THIS BOOK WAS A LABOR OF LOVE FOR ME, BUT IT WOULD have never been possible without the support of an army of people.

First and foremost, thanks to my amazing family. To Ralph, my husband, who supports and takes care of me through all my crazy ideas like writing a book while I am working full time and traveling for presentations. Thanks to my amazing children, Jessica and Jacob, who both encouraged me to write this book and helped as early readers. I admire all that you both do in life.

Thanks to the friends and classmates who weathered the storm of medical school with me and to my fellow dermatology residents who made learning about skin fun.

Thank you to all my many mentors over the years. Thanks to those mentors I have mentioned in this book as well as those who were not mentioned. From Friends Select School in Philadelphia to medical school at the University of Pennsylvania and residency at the University of Michigan, there have so many who helped shape and support me. Thanks to the mentors at Wake Forest University School of Medicine, both inside and outside of my department for encouraging my leadership journey. I say a warm thank you to my first friend at Wake Forest School of Medicine, Dr. Brenda Latham-Sadler, who has paved the way for so many Black, indigenous, and people of color in medical school.

Thanks to my many friends and colleagues who have been on the diversity champion journey with me and who inspire me every day with all that they do.

Thanks to those who reviewed and helped strengthen the book: Dr. Ronata Hall (my sister-in-law and overall wise person), Dr. Lindsay Strowd (my colleague, friend, and chair), Dr. Victoria Barbosa (dermatology colleague and diversity champion), and Dr. Kayla Taylor (mentee and dermatology resident). You all helped me galvanize my ideas and improve my message.

Thank you to Dr. Shani Smith, my mentee, friend, and colleague, who brought tears to my eyes with the heartfelt foreword that she wrote for this book.

Thank you to my lovely, kind, and magical writing coach, Azul Terronez, at Authors Who Lead. He and his team at Mandala Tree Press were so helpful in getting the words on the page to form a cohesive message while making sure the final product looks like a beautiful treat.

And finally, thanks to my many mentees for trusting me to help to guide their medical careers.

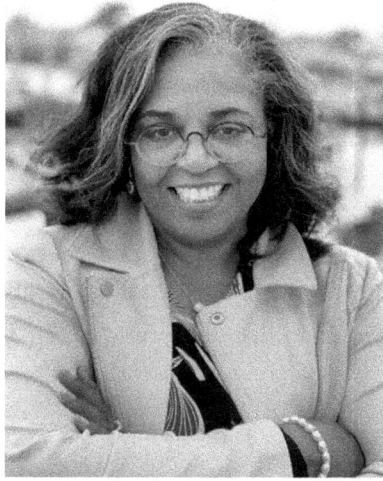

About the Author

Dr. Amy McMichael is a Philadelphia native who received her medical degree from the University of Pennsylvania School of Medicine and completed her dermatology residency at the University of Michigan School of Medicine.

She is a professor in the Department of Dermatology at Wake Forest School of Medicine in Winston-Salem, NC, and has held leadership positions in the department for over twenty years. She was residency program director for twelve years and then was chair of the department for eleven years. After stepping down as chair in 2022, she continues to wear many hats as a clinician, researcher, and teacher.

Her passion is mentorship, and she has formally mentored over thirty-five students, residents, and young physicians and informally mentored more than one hundred learners at all levels of education. She spends 20 percent of her personal time counselling those who are interested in medicine and dermatology.

When she is not working and mentoring, she enjoys reading, traveling, and spending time with her family and friends. This is her first nonfiction book, which grew out of her many inspiring interactions with students, residents, and early career physicians.

I would appreciate your feedback on what chapters helped you most and what you would like to see in future books.

If you enjoyed this book and found it helpful, please leave a review on Amazon.

Visit me at

DERMDOWNLOAD.COM

where you can sign up for email updates.

THANK YOU!

www.ingramcontent.com/pod-product-compliance
Lightning Source LLC
Chambersburg PA
CBHW060133100426
42744CB00007B/772